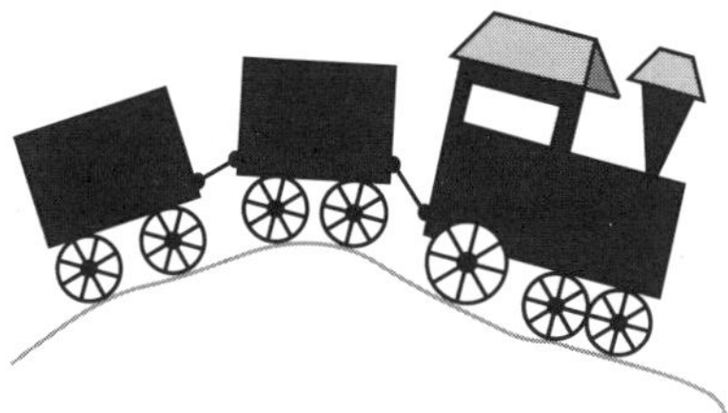

Headed Home:
Developmental Intervention for Hospitalized Infants and Their Families

Kathy S. Katz, Ph.D.
Child Development Center
Georgetown University Medical Center
Washington, D.C.

with Chapter Contributions from

Deborah P. Osborn, RN, Ed.M.,
Cynthia Baker, MA, Kathleen A. Shapiro, P.T.,
and Sharon Willig, M.A., SLP-CCC

Published by:
VORT Corporation
Palo Alto, CA 94306

Printed in the United States of America.

Published by:
VORT Corporation
PO Box 60132
Palo Alto, CA 94306

ISBN 0-89718-122-0

Publisher's Note

We are pleased to have the opportunity to publish this important resource. It is concise and comprehensive, yet we cannot anticipate the circumstances under which a reader may apply its contents. Each child is unique and masters skills and develops at a rate and an age often different from other children. We therefore urge that you seek additional professional advice if you have any concerns about a child's health or development. We expressly decline liability for the results of conclusions you may reach about a child after reading and applying the contents of this book.

Table of Contents

Acknowledgments

This guide is the product of the joint efforts of a large number of professionals and families. We would like to acknowledge the contribution of Project Headed Home staff members who assisted in the development of the clinical service model. These include Janeece Warfield, Psy.D., Anne Crawford, RN, Maureen Reilly, M.S.N., CPNP, Suzanne Baptista, P.T., and our infant specialist/illustrator, Dani L. Rusnak, Ed.M.

We are grateful for the warm reception offered to the project by Carolyn Parry, RN, PICU Nursing Coordinator, the nursing staff, and the PICU medical staff, including Gabriel Hauser, MD, and Yolande Smith, MD. The cardiology medical specialists and the cardiology nurse specialists, Marilyn Clare, RN, and Jeanne Ricks, RN, freely offered us many hours of information sessions about the implications of cardiac disease for developmental functioning.

Transcription and editing of the manuscript were provided by Elka Booth, whose good humor and multiple talents were of immeasurable support to the Project. Thanks for patience and understanding go to our own families, especially to Dick, Marisa and Eliza, and to John and Delaney. Most especially, we would like to express our gratitude to the families participating in Project Headed Home, who allowed us to share in and learn from both the joyous and tragic experiences that are an integral part of life with a chronically ill child.

Partial support for this guide was provided through a Handicapped Children's Early Education Program grant (HO24F80025) from the U.S. Department of Education, Office of Special Education Programs to the Georgetown University Child Development Center.

Chapter 1

Trends in Management of Chronically Ill Children

Kathy S. Katz, Ph.D.

The increased survival rate of premature infants in the last decade has been at the cost of an increase in the number of children who survive with chronic medical conditions. Improved surgical interventions also have contributed to longer survival of children with congenital abnormalities. Numbers of these children remain dependent on medical technology and require lengthy hospitalization before discharge. Many more remain medically fragile, requiring skilled nursing or frequent rehospitalizations at periods of time (Koop, 1983).

In the past, children with chronic medical needs requiring nursing care were usually managed in institutional settings designed for chronic care. In recent years, chronically ill children have other options for care, including small group nursing settings and home-based care. The result is that these children remain within the community and thus require a variety of support services. However, periodic illness results in rehospitalization on a frequent basis. In order for the needs of these children to be served, professionals in both hospital and community settings must be familiar with strategies to maximize good developmental outcome.

CONTRIBUTIONS TO THE EXPANDED MOVE TOWARDS HOME CARE

The current approach to care for chronically ill children is consistent with contemporary philosophy towards care for individuals with other types of disabilities. Instead of institutional care, disabled individuals have more options for residing in community settings available to them.

A number of factors underlie this philosophical change. In the past it was perhaps felt that institutional settings offered advantages in terms of a wide range of services to maximize progress. The variety of available medical personnel and the range of technological equipment served to make the hospital seem the best environment for a child who remained medically fragile. Current concerns about the deleterious effects of prolonged institutional care on development have resulted in more alternatives being sought to *normalize the environment* of the chronically ill child, to the extent possible. *Technological advances* are among the factors that have made home care a viable alternative to institutional care. The development of portable ventilators, home dialysis, and monitoring alarm systems are examples of available technology that make home care management possible (Kohrman, in press).

Growth in home care management has also resulted from the greater *advocacy* roles parents have assumed for their children and themselves. Medical plans may now be developed in keeping with *family needs* and goals rather than in addressing the child in isolation from the family system. Long-term hospitalization may have negative affects on the child and may contribute to the prolonged stress on a family which is trying to maintain a relationship with their hospitalized child. While the stresses of maintaining a chronically ill child in the home setting may be great, for some families these may be preferable to those experienced during hospitalization.

Perhaps the most significant impact on expansion of home care has been that *cost effectiveness* has been demonstrated in maintaining a chronically ill child at home rather than in a chronic care facility. Despite the variety of support services a medically fragile child requires at home, these costs will still usually be greatly exceeded by the cost of acute hospitalization even in intermediate care facilities (Kettrick, 1983). For youngsters whose cases are very complex, however, the costs of setting up a "mini" Intensive Care Unit at home may, in fact, exceed those of providing the same services in the institutional unit . The cost factor is not a valid argument for home care in these cases. However, this is not to say that other benefits of home care don't outweigh cost differences.

IMPACT ON FAMILIES

The move towards home care of chronically ill children was spearheaded by parents of these children. For many families, the complicated preparations and daily anxieties of home care are outweighed by having their family intact. But the compromises families must make to maintain their children at home are many.

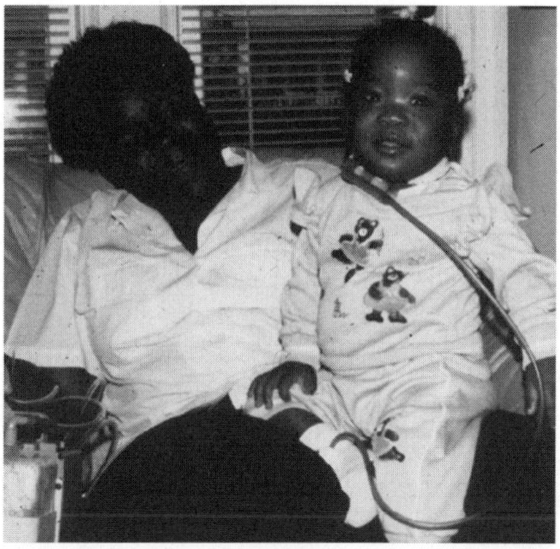

The *dependence on the technological equipment* is often stressful for families. It is sometimes difficult to perceive the child as other than an extension of the equipment necessary to keep him or her alive (Kohrman, in press). Equipment maintenance is a continual chore; malfunctions are common. For the ventilator-dependent child, malfunction and power loss are major threats to survival. Backup arrangements must be in place to protect against such occurrence (Goldberg et al., 1984).

For those families not provided home nursing services, difficulties in finding qualified alternative caregivers are frequently experienced. While *opportunities for respite* from the continuous caretaking burden are felt to be essential for families providing home care, these are often expensive or difficult to secure. Problems with finding alternative caregivers, combined with hesitation on the part of some friends to become involved with the prolonged stress associated with care for the chronically ill child, may result in a sense of *social isolation* for the family. Friends, who early on offered support, often begin to distance themselves. The family may find their social relationships confined primarily to other families of chronically ill children, or to the professional staff providing services.

The caregiving burden usually falls most heavily on *mothers*. It is not uncommon for women to feel that they must give up jobs, despite financial hardship, because of the need to be available for the ill child. *Fathers* may feel trapped into jobs from which they would ordinarily advance, but with which they must remain either because of lack of freedom to move from a geographic area, or fears of jeopardizing insurance coverage with any change in employment (Feinberg, 1985). *Siblings* may also have to assume responsibilities not usually expected of their peers. Their needs often come second to the persistent needs of the ill child. Some siblings respond to these pressures with a grave maturity. Others may show disruptive behavior at home or school which is reflective of their emotional stress (Peck, 1986).

The unpredictable nature of the ill child's health makes long-range planning difficult. Often, plans for much needed family vacations must be scrapped because of sudden acute illness of the child. Some families are able to handle these pressures and have a tremendous sense of sharing that brings the family together. Not all families can achieve this.

Other families may be terrified of the responsibilities assumed in caring for a chronically ill child at home. *Professionals must be cautious not to let their personal biases about care settings for these children put pressure on families into selecting or rejecting home care for themselves.* Contemporary trends for home care may put undue stress on families who do not feel able to assume these responsibilities. For these families, other options for intermediate care are available in many areas. While certainly not equivalent to a home setting, some of these facilities have incorporated infant and early childhood development programs into their medical caregiving plans. Some families must be reassured that the needs of the family as a whole may outweigh the needs of the ill child in family decision-making (Katz et al., 1989).

FINANCIAL SUPPORT FOR HOME CARE

Demonstration that, in many instances, home care of chronically ill children can be less expensive than prolonged inpatient care has produced more options for financial support of home-based care (Goldberg et al., 1984). While insurance programs vary greatly in their policies towards home-based service reimbursement, if it can be demonstrated that a cost saving exists, some plans are willing to adjust reimbursement procedures. This may be particularly true of health maintenance plans. Less flexible insurance companies continue to require costly inpatient services in order for coverage to be provided.

Because of the persistent efforts of parents, such as those of Katie Beckett, who sought to win acceptance for home-based coverage for services for their chronically ill child, many states now provide state-supported coverage for home-based care. This reimbursement policy involves a waiver for use of Medicaid reimbursement for services that were previously paid for only if provided in hospitals. Despite the strides made in improved funding for home-based care, arranging such funding is often a monumental task. To make it possible usually takes a combination of public, private and personal financing.

Whether new resources may yet be made available to support some aspects of home-based care remains a possibility with the advent of Public Law 99-457. This legislation, more recently updated as the Individuals with Disabilities Education Act (IDEA) Part H, is designed to provide incentives to states to offer early intervention services to disabled and at-risk children from birth to three years of age. While the legislation is not designed to support medical services per se, some of the educational and allied health services required by chronically ill children may be covered (Sciarillo et al., 1988). This legislation's emphasis on family-focused intervention is also an aspect of the intervention model that may provide particular support to families of chronically ill children. The intent of this legislation is that intervention will target needs as the family identifies them and that these needs may go beyond those of the child, himself. Thus, if families determine that counseling for a sibling is an important part of the intervention plan for the chronically ill child, it is possible that this type of service might be provided. The IDEA Part H legislation is a potentially valuable support that may allow more families to manage a chronically ill child at home (McGonigel et al., 1991).

NEEDS DURING HOSPITALIZATION

While chronically ill infants are now being managed more regularly at home, they often continue to require frequent *rehospitalizations.* These occur in conjunction with episodes of acute illness that require more intensive medical care.

These episodes are *disruptive* to both child and family. The family must once again juggle being available at the hospital for the ill child and keeping up with the needs of the rest of the household. Acute illness of the child may again raise the spectre of death. Parents must cope with the uncertainty of whether their child will live through the latest crisis.

For the child, acute illness may mean *setbacks* in growth and developmental progress that had been so hard won. It is not unusual to see a child lose recently attained skills for a period following illness. This may be frustrating for the child and discouraging for her family. While a continued emphasis during hospitalization on developmental goals is highly desirable, the child may not be able to participate actively in beneficial activities when she is sickest. Medical/nursing caregivers in the hospital have only in recent years become aware of strategies for maintaining a developmental program for the child during hospitalization. Early interventionists may be helpful in familiarizing hospital staff with techniques to incorporate developmental goals into medical care plans. Some strategies do not require active participation from the child but provide her with particular positions or sensory exposure that may be beneficial.

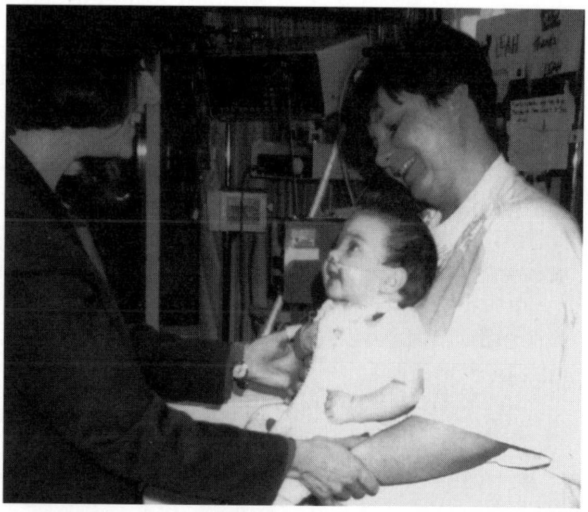

The increased survival of chronically ill children means that more of these children will be going home to live in the community. However, it also means that these children will return to an inpatient status at times with needs quite different from the usually healthy child hospitalized with an acute illness, such as pneumonia. Hospital personnel will need to be increasingly knowledgeable about management strategies for chronically ill children during hospitalization, addressing both medical and developmental needs. They will also have to be sensitive to the needs of the child's family as a whole in order to help them through the hospitalization experience.

Lastly, hospital personnel will be challenged to expand their knowledge of the variety of support services available to the child's family when she returns home. Hospital staff are already familiar with medically related services in the community. They must now gain enhanced awareness of the early intervention resources available so that both medical and developmental needs can be addressed simultaneously with the child at home.

NEEDS IN THE COMMUNITY

With greater numbers of chronically ill children headed home from the hospital to the community, more community-based resource personnel will be called upon to serve a population with whom they have previously had little contact. Many early childhood educators have not had experience working with medically fragile children. The medical status of the child may be frightening or overwhelming for the educator. Many center-based infant intervention or daycare programs have not previously had to enroll chronically ill young children. There may be resistance in accepting the responsibility of having the chronically ill child participate in the program. However, with the right preparation of staff in these programs, chronically ill children can participate successfully without detriment to their health status or undue stress to the staff. Much planning and training must occur first for this to happen.

PURPOSE OF THE GUIDE

The issues discussed in this chapter are those currently being grappled with in efforts to meet the needs of chronically ill children and their families. This guide was designed to assist both health care providers and early intervention personnel in developing knowledge and skills to meet these needs.

The major emphasis of this guide is on provision of services during hospitalization and in transition to home care. While a body of literature exists on developmental intervention with prematures in the NICU, little has been described for inpatient programming for older infants and their families. These children are usually rehospitalized in the Pediatric Intensive Care Unit (PICU) or on the General Pediatric Ward. The chronically ill child is often considered a "regular" on the floor because of the frequency or length of his hospitalizations. While the medical needs of this group of children have been remarkably well met with current medical technology, their developmental needs have often been overlooked because of pressing medical concerns. Similarly, the child's needs have been the primary focus of the care plan, sometimes with little regard for how this might fit into the family situation. Current approaches to management of chronically ill children during hospitalization have attempted to incorporate broader goals into the care plan.

Subsequent chapters of this guide will provide an overview of the developmental intervention goals to be considered and specific activities that can be introduced to enhance development in chronically ill children. Assisting families in coping with hospitalizations and preparing them for home management is a critical role for professionals serving chronically ill infants. This guide places a major emphasis on supporting families caring for chronically ill children. Current attitudes on the parent-professional relationship reflect an increased partnership in planning and decision-making around the needs of the child. The development of this approach to service delivery will be reviewed.

Professionals working with hospitalized infants may be interested in learning about a specific program that might be adapted to their own facility. The demonstration program, "Project Headed Home" of Georgetown University, will be described. This interdisciplinary program incorporates many of the recommended procedures for providing exemplary care to chronically ill infants and their families.

It is hoped that in the coming years, as medical technology continues to prolong life for chronically ill children, that developmental knowledge will have made similar strides. Professionals serving this population need to be aware of intervention strategies to enhance developmental outcome for the child. They must also be knowledgeable about methods for providing family support to meet the challenges of caring for a chronically ill child.

REFERENCES

Feinberg, E. (1985). Family stress in pediatric home care. *Caring, 6,* 38-41.

Goldberg, A., Faure, E., Vaugh, C., Snarski, R., & Seleny, F. (1984). Home care for life supported persons: An approach to program development. *Journal of Pediatrics, 104;* 785-795.

McGonigel, M., Kaufmann, R., & Johnson, B. (1991). *Guidelines and recommended practices for the individualized family service plan* (2nd ed.) Bethesda, MD: Association for the Care of Children's Health.

Katz, K., Pokorni, J., & Long, T. (1989). *Chronically ill and at risk infants: Family-centered intervention from hospital to home.* Palo Alto: VORT Corporation.

Kettrick, R. (1983). Programs for the care of ventilator dependent children: The Pennsylvania program. In *Report of the Surgeon General's workshop on children with handicaps and their families.* DHHS Publication #PHS83-50194, Washington, DC: U.S. Department of Health and Human Services.

Kohrman, A. (in press). Psychological issues in pediatric home care. In M. Mehlman & S. Younger. *Issues in high technology home care: A guide for decision-making.*

Koop, E. (1983). *Report of the Surgeon General's workshop on children with handicaps and their families.* DHHS Publication #PHS83-50194, Washington, DC: U.S. Department of Health and Human Services.

Peck, T. (1986). Siblings of chronically ill children. In E. Ahmann (Ed.), *Home care for the high risk infant.* Rockville, MD: Aspen Publications.

Sciarillo, W., Draper, S., Green, P., Burkett, K., & Demetrides, S. (1988). Children with specialized health needs in the special education setting. A statewide technical assistance approach. *Infants and Young Children, 1,* 74-84.

Chapter 2

Medical Needs of Chronically Ill Infants

Deborah Powell Osborn, RN, Ed.M.

Technological advances over the past 20 years have brought enormous change in the way our society cares for the chronically ill child. In the past, trained medical professionals cared for chronically ill children in hospital settings. More recently, these very same children, some of whom require mechanical ventilation, dialysis and intravenous therapy, receive care in the home from family and staff from community-based agencies, most of whom have had little or no formal medical training. Increasingly, educators, physical therapists and speech-language therapists are becoming responsible for providing services for children who are medically fragile. This may contribute to anxiety for professionals not trained in the management of chronic illness. This chapter will discuss some of these chronic conditions, their associated technologies, the relevant medical considerations for early interventionists, and strategies to improve communication between family members and professionals.

The chronic medical conditions of infancy are so numerous that it is beyond the scope of this chapter to provide a comprehensive listing. Instead, a few of the major chronic conditions that are commonly found in children who are referred to early intervention programs have been chosen for discussion. These are further divided into two categories:

- Medical conditions associated with prematurity
- Chronic conditions found in full-term infants

The intent of this chapter is to familiarize the early interventionist with these disease processes so that he or she will feel confident in serving chronically ill infants.

MEDICAL CONDITIONS ASSOCIATED WITH PREMATURITY

The medical conditions associated with prematurity occur primarily as a result of the immaturity of the infant's organ systems at delivery and secondarily, due to the invasive treatments and technologies necessary to maintain the infant's life. Premature infants may encounter difficulties with every major organ system at one time or another, including cardiorespiratory, neurologic, and gastrointestinal. The following discussion will highlight the medical conditions commonly found in premature infants that may result in chronic illness.

Bronchopulmonary Dysplasia

One of the most common forms of chronic lung disease in infants born prematurely is bronchopulmonary dysplasia (BPD). Since it was first described in 1967 (Northway and his associates), its incidence has risen due to the increasing survival rate of ever smaller preterm infants.

The specific cause of BPD remains unclear. However, it is believed that the major factors contributing to BPD are:

- Exposure to high concentrations of oxygen
- The use of positive pressure ventilation for prolonged periods of time
- Immaturity of the lung structure
- Endotracheal intubation

The combination of these factors leads to detrimental changes in the infant's airway, which may include the following:

- Increased mucous production
- Paralyzed cilia, resulting in a decreased ability to remove mucous
- Limited alveolar growth, resulting in increased need for oxygen

(Bozynski, 1989)

Though lung development continues after birth, thus improving the prognosis for many children, this development is compromised by the very treatment that is necessary for sustaining life. Moreover, the extent of permanent lung damage is difficult to predict; some infants with BPD will sustain damage too severe to sustain life.

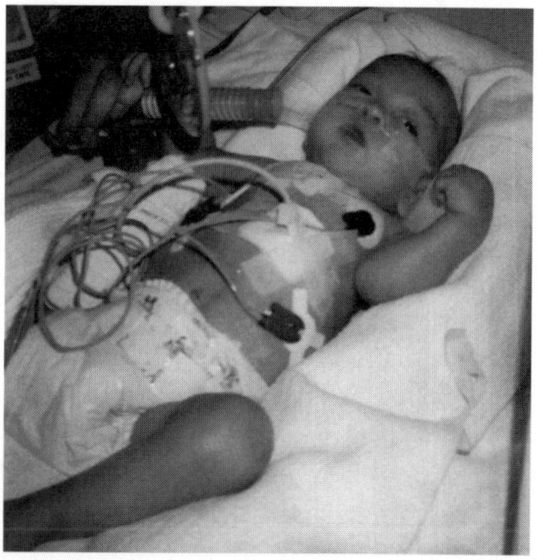

For those infants who do survive, their pulmonary status remains limited and they are more susceptible to respiratory infection in the early years. However, by the time they reach school age, the majority achieve relatively normal lung function (Ensher & Clark, 1986).

The clinical signs of children with BPD vary depending upon the severity of lung damage. An increased respiratory rate (tachypnea) and respiratory distress (barrel chest, nasal flaring, and chest retractions) are the most common findings in infants with BPD. Other medical complications associated with BPD and/or its therapy include:

- Cyanotic (blue) spells
- Osteopenia (fragile, poorly mineralized bones)
- Hypertension
- Kidney stones
- Central airway narrowing or weakness (tracheal stenosis, tracheomalacia)
- Congestive heart failure
- Gastroesophageal reflux
- Poor growth
- Feeding problems

(Bozynski, 1989)

Early intervention professionals need to be aware of the various complications or problems associated with BPD in order to provide appropriate therapy. For example, infants with BPD remain at risk for recurrent respiratory infections. Every fall and winter many children with BPD are admitted to the hospital with respiratory infections such as Respiratory Syncytial Virus (RSV). RSV is a common viral infection from which a healthy infant rapidly recovers but which may be life-threatening for infants with BPD. For this reason early interventionists should be cognizant of preliminary signs and symptoms of respiratory infections in the children in their program, as well as themselves, and take care to prevent the spread of infection among their clients. These signs would include:

- A change in secretions
- A change in respiratory pattern or rate
- Irritability
- Loss of appetite

Children who have required prolonged mechanical ventilation are at risk for chronic otitis media (ear infections) which may cause conductive hearing loss. Again, it is imperative that the interventionist be alert to early signs, including fever without apparent congestion, pulling on the ears, failing to respond to noise, and waking from sleep in apparent pain, and then refer for appropriate evaluation and treatment.

In instances of BPD associated with gastroesophageal reflux (GE reflux), poor growth, or feeding problems, an early interventionist may reduce symptoms through positioning techniques, and specific feeding techniques described in Chapter 5. Infants with severe BPD will have increased caloric requirements but an intolerance of large fluid volumes or formula with high caloric density, making it difficult to maintain adequate nutrition. This may be further affected by irritability, vomiting and gastroesophageal reflux. Other feeding problems associated with BPD include poor tolerance in the introduction of textured foods and spoon feeding.

Technology needs associated with BPD vary greatly from child to child. In the most severe case an infant discharged from the hospital to home may require mechanical ventilation, tracheostomy care, nebulizer treatments, chest therapy, suctioning, various medications, oxygen saturation monitor, apnea monitor, and skilled nursing care. In less severe cases, children who are discharged may require low-flow oxygen delivered by nasal cannula, monitoring devices, chest physiotherapy, nebulizer treatments, and a variety of medications. More fortunate children may be sent home requiring no additional technologies at all. To provide appropriate therapy for the infant and support to the parents, the interventionist must be comfortable in working with infants who require various medical and technological supports.

Children with tracheostomies present particular difficulties for interventionists, although not because interventionists are expected to provide nursing care. Rather, they must be aware of the medical consequences and risks that result from having a trach and the extent to which such consequences and risks will affect the interventionists' interaction with the children.

A tracheostomy is surgically created if a child requires long-term ventilation or if the child's tracheal airway is small due to multiple intubations. The parents or caregivers of the child must be trained to perform both routine and emergency care procedures associated with the trach. The procedures include:

- Maintaining the proper equipment and supplies
- Maintaining a source of humidity
- Suctioning tracheal secretions
- Removing and cleaning the inner cannula daily
- Routine inspection of trach site
- Changing the tracheostomy tie daily
- Changing the entire trach tube on a regular basis
- Providing emergency care (including CPR) when needed

Interventionists need not be fully cognizant of all caregiving techniques associated with the above procedures, but they should be aware of the possible complications associated with a tracheostomy. Interventionists should be aware, at a minimum, of the necessity of suctioning the tracheostomy on a regular basis to ensure an open airway free of secretions and mucous. A child's need to be suctioned is not always predictable; therefore, an interventionist untrained in suctioning should not be left alone with a trached child, but should know when to summon assistance for purposes of suctioning. As Ahmann (1986) notes, the following are indications that a child needs to be suctioned:

- Secretions can be heard bubbling in the airway
- Breath sounds are dry and wheezing
- Child complains of difficulty breathing
- Child has fast breathing not caused by activity
- Child has signs of low oxygen, such as restlessness, fast heart rate, flaring of the nostrils, blue or dusky color around the mouth or nose

Interventionists should also be aware of the effects that the tracheostomy has on an infant's activities of daily life. Most children with a tracheostomy can eat and drink without difficulty, but vomiting may occur when the infant attempts to cough up secretions during or after feedings, or when suctioned during or after feedings. Therefore, before you begin feeding a child with a trach, request that the child be suctioned, and do not suction again until two hours after the child has eaten. Brief and gentle suctioning should be used if it is necessary to suction during or shortly after a meal.

Bathing (or water play) need not be restricted just because the child has a tracheostomy. Infants and children should be carefully monitored to avoid getting water into the tracheostomy, but there is no reason to avoid bathing or allowing the child to play at a water table.

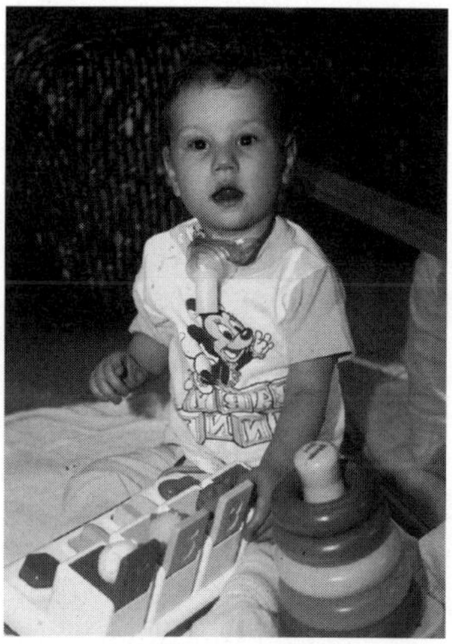

The child with a tracheostomy is at risk for developing communication problems and should therefore receive treatment from a speech-language pathologist as soon as possible. This risk stems from several factors. Often the child's need to communicate is minimal due to the excessive attention he or she receives from medical and caregiving personnel. In addition, the presence of a tracheostomy tube in the upper airway can inhibit the passage of air through the glottis which causes aphonia or the inability to produce voice. Additional factors causing the lack of vocalization include:

- Use of a ventilator
- Weakened respiratory muscles
- Poor diaphragmatic movements

(Simon, 1986)

Infants and children with tracheostomies need not be housebound. Parents, for their mental health as well as their child's, should be encouraged to get out of the house. But families must remember that certain supplies must always accompany the child with a tracheostomy on short or long trips. They include:

- Trach tube with ties in place
- Trach tube which is one size smaller

- Bandage scissors
- Portable suction
- Saline
- Tissues
- Ambu bag

(Ahmann, 1986)

Finally, when the child travels in a car, two adults should always accompany the child, one to drive the car and their other to attend to the child. Interventionists should encourage parents to take their child out of the house, and they can assist them by providing needed support.

Cerebral Insults

Intraventricular hemorrhage and periventricular leukomalacia are two common types of cerebral insults associated with prematurity. Both can have devastating effects on the child and his subsequent development.

Intraventricular Hemorrhage

The blood vessels in the germinal matrix area of the brain in premature infants are relatively fragile and susceptible to breakage and bleeding in the event of too little or too much blood flow. The infant's immature auto-regulatory mechanisms may fail to control cerebral blood flow resulting in intraventricular hemorrhage (IVH) (Vaucher, 1988).

Before neuroimaging was possible, IVH was believed to be an infrequent, though usually fatal, complication of preterm birth. Studies using ultrasound and CAT scans now show that IVH occurs in approximately 40 percent to 45 percent of all preterm infants, with most bleeds occurring in the first three to four days after birth. The incidence and severity of hemorrhage is related to the degree of prematurity, with the smallest (<1,250 grams) and most immature (<30 weeks gestation) infants at a greater risk for the most severe degree of bleeding (Vaucher, 1988).

Intraventricular hemorrhages are classified by their size, amount of blood in the ventricular system, and whether there is brain tissue (intraparenchymal) involvement. Such hemorrhages are classified by grade in increasing severity, as follows:

- Grade I - Small amount of bleeding flows into the lining over ventricles
- Grade II - Blood partially fills but does not dilate the ventricles
- Grade III - Both ventricles are filled and dilated with blood
- Grade IV - Bleeding extends from the ventricles into the adjacent brain tissue

(Vaucher, 1988)

A positive correlation exists between the severity of the hemorrhage and the occurrence of neurologic complications. The most frequent complication found in infants surviving severe IVH (Grade III-IV) is hydrocephalus (Pettett, 1986). Some infants with post-hemorrhagic hydrocephalus will eventually require a solution to control increasing intraventricular pressure. Permanent control of intraventricular pressure is accomplished by the diversion of cerebrospinal fluid by means of the surgical placement of a ventriculoperitoneal (VP) shunt (i.e., carrying the fluid from the ventricle or the brain into the abdominal cavity). Shunt obstruction and infection remain potential lifelong problems for these infants. Care providers need to be alert to signs of obstruction or infection which are discussed later in this chapter.

Long-term follow-up studies of IVH patients indicate that the severity of neurodevelopmental problems is related to the severity of the hemorrhage. While small amounts of intraventricular bleeding are not associated with an increased risk of major neurodevelopmental problems, some studies have demonstrated subtle deficits (perceptual-motor, verbal, quantitative and memory) that become apparent at school age. However, the incidence of cerebral palsy and mental retardation is clearly higher in those children with more severe hemorrhage, such as a Grade III or Grade IV, with some studies suggesting a 50-75 percent chance of handicap (Vaucher, 1988).

Periventricular Leukomalacia

Periventricular leukomalacia (PVL), also called periventricular echodensities (PVE), is yet another type of cerebral injury associated with prematurity which often results in long-term disability in the child. PVL is the loss of cell tissue surrounding the ventricles, which occurs as a result of a lack of blood and oxygen to susceptible areas of the brain. The most common site of white matter injury is close to the region of brain responsible for vision and motor control. Damage to the white matter in this area results most often in cerebral palsy, frequently in conjunction with cortical visual deficits. Infants who have experienced this loss of white matter may appear asymptomatic in the first few months of life, even when fairly extensive areas are involved, but there has not been associated hemorrhage and increased intraventricular pressure. PVL may, therefore, not be recognized unless carefully evaluated through ultrasound scan (Vaucher, 1988).

Interventionists should note that, as with intraventricular hemorrhage, the neurodevelopmental outcome is variable in infants with PVL, depending on the size and location of the injury. However, PVL is even more frequently associated with adverse neuromotor outcomes (i.e., cerebral palsy) than is IVH (Vaucher, 1988).

VISION DEFICITS

Blindness has been recognized as a serious consequence of prematurity since 1954, when a multi-center collaborative study reported that the blindness was associated with the use of high concentrations of oxygen. Subsequent capability for monitoring oxygen concentration for treating respiratory distress with premature infants was associated with a decline in the incidence of blindness (Pettett, 1986).

The term, Retinopathy of Prematurity (ROP), previously termed "retrolental fibroplasia," is used to refer to the condition that causes blindness in premature infants. Today it is believed that ROP is not caused exclusively by the administration of oxygen. Rather, the damage emerges when there is an increase in both the blood oxygen and carbon dioxide levels in particularly susceptible infants (Ensher & Clark, 1986.) ROP is divided into four stages of classification to describe the various changes that take place in the premature infant's eye. The stages of ROP are determined by a trained medical professional, usually a pediatric ophthalmologist, upon examination of the retina. The stages include:

- Stage I - Constriction of retinal blood vessels followed by abnormal growth of the vessels
- Stage II - Hemorrhaging into the retina which may or may not form scar tissue
- Stage III - Proliferation of blood vessels into the vitreous humor, with or without localized retina detachment
- Stage IV - Complete detachment of retina and then total blindness

Approximately one out of six premature infants who require oxygen develop some degree of ROP. Less than half of these infants go on to experience some visual impairment resulting from scarring. The degree of visual impairment that results depends upon the amount of scarring and the extent to which the scar tissue damages the retina. The specific visual impairments resulting from scarring and partial detachment range from myopia (near-sightedness) to loss of part of the visual field. Total blindness occurs relatively rarely (Harrison, 1983).

As with many other complications resulting from prematurity, the very small premature infants (<1000 grams) are more likely to develop eye damage than the larger preterm infants. It is estimated that 22 percent to 42 percent of these very small premature infants will suffer some type of visual impairment from ROP and that 5 percent to 11 percent will suffer permanent blindness. In comparison, only 2 percent of the infants with birthweights between 1000-1500 grams will develop eye damage, and only 0.3 percent to 1 percent will suffer blindness (Harrison, 1983).

Experimental treatments available to premature infants to lessen the severity of the disease include large doses of vitamin E in hopes of reducing susceptibility to eye damage and innovative surgical treatments using lasers or cryotherapy to help prevent total retinal detachment and blindness (Harrison, 1983).

Interventionists working with infants with a history of ROP should observe the infant's visual development and acuity and encourage the family to seek follow-up by a pediatric ophthalmologist after the infant's discharge.

SHORT BOWEL SYNDROME

Premature infants are also susceptible to gastrointestinal disorders which in severe forms can lead to death and/or chronic malabsorption problems. Necrotizing enterocolitis (NEC) and short bowel syndrome are two such conditions. NEC is a destructive infection of the small bowel occurring shortly after the introduction of the first oral feeding. The immaturity of the premature infant's digestive system, combined with an increased vulnerability to tissue injury imposed by oxygen and circulation difficulties, can lead to NEC. In its milder forms NEC can be managed with medications and supportive measures during the acute phases. In its more severe forms, surgery is required to remove the damaged portion of bowel. This type of surgery also typically requires a temporary ileostomy, a surgically created connection through the abdominal wall. After some months of healing and growth, another surgical procedure can usually be performed to restore a normal passageway through the colon and rectum (Ichord, 1986). But regardless of whether or not any intestine is removed, the infant with NEC will permanently lose some length of functional intestine.

When part of the intestinal tract is removed, short bowel or gut syndrome results. Historically, children with intestinal tracts too short for adequate nutrition did not often survive. However, with advanced diagnostic and surgical techniques and total parenteral nutrition (TPN), survival rates and prognoses for such children are much improved (Gantt & Thompson, 1985).

Short bowel syndrome diminishes the infant's ability to digest a regular diet and is characterized by diarrhea, abdominal discomfort, and malnutrition. The degree of successful bowel adaptation depends on the extent and site of the intestinal loss; the surgeon will therefore attempt to preserve as much bowel as possible.

Maintaining optimal nutritional support until the intestine heals is the primary goal in caring for a child with short bowel syndrome. Nutritional support will be accomplished by:

- Selecting and providing the appropriate formula

- Treating diarrhea and skin breakdown
- Monitoring calories, nutrients, fluids and electrolytes
- Maintaining a subclavian line for TPN and intralipids until the bowel can tolerate total oral feeding
- Preventing infection

(Gantt & Thompson, 1985)

A dangerous source of infection for the infant with short bowel syndrome is the central line used for TPN. This line is a surgically placed catheter which runs into the subclavian vein. In such cases, infection may result from bacterial contamination during daily fluid and tubing changes, dressing change, or from leaks or breaks in the catheter, fluid bags, or tubing. Broviac catheters are preferred for long-term use because the tubing in this type of catheter reduces the risk of bacteria to travel along it. In addition to central line infection, infants with short bowel syndrome are prone to gastroenteritis. Because the shortened bowel no longer has normal amounts of flora, it is easily overgrown with bacteria. Diarrhea may occur and the infant may need to be taken off oral feeding to rest the bowel for several days. Once diarrhea slows, feedings may be resumed gradually (Gantt & Thompson, 1985).

As with infants with BPD, infants with chronic GI problems can suffer major setbacks from even the minor diseases of infancy. A simple intestinal virus can lead to rapid dehydration with a need for rehospitalization, and a prolonged recovery time to regain an acceptable growth rate.

CHRONIC CONDITIONS FOUND IN FULL-TERM INFANTS

It is estimated that 10 percent to 15 percent of the children in the United States have some form of chronic health impairment, the majority of which are unrelated to prematurity. Fortunately, many of these chronic conditions are mild and can be managed effectively by family physicians, pediatricians, or nurses with the occasional guidance of medical specialists (Hobbs, Perrin & Ireys, 1985). On the other hand, there are many chronic illnesses that are quite severe and require the care of a variety of specialists, sophisticated technology, and long-term or recurrent hospitalization. Despite medical advances, the number of children suffering from chronic health conditions has not reduced appreciably. This is attributable to the fact that modern medicine has allowed children who in the past would not have lived to survive for longer periods despite their chronic conditions.

For practicality, those conditions that are most typical in full-term infants followed by early intervention programs will be highlighted.

CONGENITAL HEART DEFECTS

The function of the heart is to pump oxygen and nutrients to all the tissues in the body. In the case of physiologic, anatomic, or electrical defects, the heart is unable to effectively fulfill this function. Congenital heart defects (CHD) are structural malformations of the heart, present at birth. Serious congenital defects are often identified at birth. The newborn will demonstrate breathing difficulties and will remain a bluish color despite the administration of oxygen. Less severe defects may not be evident until months later; children with such lesser defects will often have problems gaining weight, and a heart murmur may only later be noted by a pediatrician.

The incidence of congenital heart defects has been estimated at 8 per 1000 live births. Most of the affected are full-term, appropriately grown infants of normal pregnancies. The sexes and races are equally affected; however, specific lesions may show an increased frequency in one gender. For example, coarctation of the aorta and transposition of the great vessels are more common in males; in contrast, atrial septal defects and patent ductus arteriosus are more common in females. (Behrman & Kliegman, 1990).

The most common heart defects seen in infants are presented in Table 1 (Blackman, 1984).

Table 1
Common Congenital Heart Defects

- Coarctation of the aorta - a narrowing of the aorta
- Patent ductus arteriosus (PDA) - a persistent opening of the normal fetal structure (ductus arteriosus) between the descending aorta and left pulmonary artery
- Atrial septal defect (ASD) - an opening between the two atria
- Ventricular septal defect (VSD) - an opening between the two ventricles
- Tetralogy of Fallot (TOF) - a combination of four defects: a large VSD, a large right ventricle, a misplaced aorta, and a narrowed pulmonary valve which cause unoxygenated blood to mix with oxygenated blood causing cyanosis
- Transposition of the Great Vessels (TGV) - takes several forms; the most common consists of the aorta arising from the right ventricle and the pulmonary artery arising from the left ventricle, resulting in two separate parallel circulatory systems.

In most cases, etiology of a heart defect is unknown, but genetic risk factors account for about 8 percent of cardiac defects and environmental risk factors for about 2 percent. Up to 90 percent of cardiac defects fall into a category that is described as multi-factorial (Higgins, 1987).

Approximately 30 percent of infants born with heart defects have other conditions that affect their health and development. Table 2 shows some of the genetic disorders that are frequently associated with particular heart defects. These CHD's may also occur in the absence of any genetic disorder (Behrman & Kliegman, 1990).

The impact that the defect has on the health of the child depends upon the type and severity of the defect. Minor defects that do not compromise the child, such as ASD or VSD, may not require corrective procedures unless the condition worsens markedly. Severe malformations, however, such as TGV or TOF, in which the blood bypasses the lungs, can be life-threatening. These must be treated early unless the child's immaturity or poor physical status make major corrective surgery too great a risk. In such instances, a temporary surgical procedure may be performed that provides improved oxygenation of the blood with a plan for later or final correction.

During the first years of life, children with significant heart defects may require frequent hospitalization for treatment of their heart condition as well as for various associated medical problems. The other medical problems experienced by the children in conjunction with congenital heart defects include:

- Congestive heart failure
- Failure to thrive
- Infections

Congestive heart failure (CHF) is a condition in which the heart becomes strained due to illness or fatigue and is unable to pump the blood as efficiently as it should. Inefficient pumping causes fluid to back up into the lungs, liver, and other organs.

Table 2
Congenital Heart Defects and Association with Other Conditions

Cardiac Anomaly	Syndrome
Ventricular Septal Defect (VSD)	Down Syndrome Trisomy 18 Trisomy 13 CHARGE association VATER association Holt-Oram Syndrome
Coarctation of the Aorta	Turner's Syndrome Aperts Syndrome
Patent Ductus Arteriosus (PDA)	Trisomy 18 Trisomy 13 Down Syndrome
Atrial Septal Defect (ASD)	Trisomy 18 Trisomy 13 Down Syndrome CHARGE association Holt-Oram Syndrome
Tetralogy of Fallot	CHARGE association Down Syndrome
Aortic Stenosis	Turner Syndrome Down Syndrome

The ability to recognize the cardinal signs of CHF is important for any therapist working with an infant who is at risk for developing this problem. The signs of heart failure in infants include:

- Increased respiratory rate—more than 60 breaths/minute (tachypnea)
- Labored or difficult breathing (dyspnea)
- Profuse sweating (diaphoresis)
- Wheezing
- Puffy eyelids
- Irritability
- Weak cry
- Poor sucking stamina
- Poor weight gain

If a therapist notices any change in the infant's status with respect to these symptoms, he or she should consult immediately with the parents if the child is at home, or with the medical/nursing staff, if the child is hospitalized.

Treatment for the infant with CHF is directed toward relieving respiratory distress. This can be accomplished by:

- Placing the infant in an upright posture with the use of an infant seat
- Restricting activity
- Administering oxygen
- Providing small, frequent feedings using a soft, "preemie" nipple

The following drugs may be prescribed in order to prevent and/or treat congestive heart failure:

- *Digitalis* to improve the contractablity of the heart muscle, thus allowing the heart to pump blood more efficiently
- *Diuretics* to reduce pulmonary congestion (fluid build-up in the lungs) and, if present, peripheral edema (swelling)
- *Morphine* for sedation to allow for rest in the acute stage.

Another sign of stress in a child with certain heart defects is **cyanosis** (bluish hue to skin). To avoid undue stress and fatigue on the child, interventionists should carefully monitor the infant's skin color when providing therapy for infants with certain heart defects (TOF, TGV). Increasing cyanosis may be life-threatening, so it must be recorded and reported immediately to the physician, nurse, and/or family. Cyanotic spells (hypoxic spells) are characterized by deep and rapid respirations, irritability, and worsening cyanosis. The spell may end with limpness or, if it is severe, possibly death. If such a spell should occur, the interventionist must immediately stop therapy and place the infant in a knee to chest position; this position decreases the workload of the heart.

Failure to thrive is a common problem for many infants with congenital heart defects. The poor oxygenation of blood and the increased caloric needs that accompany the most severe defects result in poor tissue growth, causing the child to be small and underdeveloped. Tube feedings are a common need for many of these children. Families will usually be instructed to:

- Limit meal times to 40 minutes.
- Provide small, frequent feedings.
- Maximize calories; offer milk or juice between feedings.
- Encourage parents to make mealtime enjoyable for the child.

(Higgins, 1987)

As with many other chronic conditions, children with congenital heart defects are prone to **infections**, particularly of the respiratory variety. Children with defects consisting of narrowed valves or holes between the heart chambers are also susceptible to bacteria growth due to inadequate circulation of the blood. In rare instances, clumps of such bacteria may break off and lodge in the brain, causing an abscess. These complications must be identified and treated with antibiotics as quickly as possible.

In summary, the management of congenital heart defects depends on the type of lesion. Some children will require only routine care, while others must receive intensive monitoring, multiple surgeries, and repeated admissions to the hospital. Interventionists working with these children should understand both the nature of the heart defect and the rationale for treatment in order to provide therapy in line with the child's physical condition. The child should be continuously monitored for signs of fatigue, cyanosis, and infection.

NEUROLOGIC DISORDERS

Neurologic disorders that affect young children can lead to a variety of developmental problems. Some neurologic disorders will make an impact upon a child's motor skills, while others will affect a child's cognitive development. The effects may vary from minimal to severe. This section will focus on the more typical neurological disorders of infants and young children.

Seizure Disorders

Seizure disorders are the most frequently occurring neurologic disorders in children; approximately 4 percent of all children experience one or more seizures between infancy and childhood (Egan & Lierman, 1986). Seizures are characterized by one or more of the following symptoms:

- Involuntary motor activity
- Unusual changes in behavior
- Change in level of consciousness

These symptoms reflect an underlying problem with normal brain functioning. In a normally functioning brain, electrical impulses travel along specific nerve pathways in a controlled manner and at appropriate times. Seizures occur when unorganized electrical bursts interfere with this normal brain function. Seizure classification is dependent upon the type of electrical bursts which occur in a particular area of the brain (Wolraich, 1984).

Wolraich (1984) describes the types of seizures typically seen in childhood; they include the following:

Infantile spasms (infantile myoclonic seizures)

- Develop between three and nine months of age
- Characterized by brief dropping of the head and flexion of the arms
- Can occur hundreds of times a day
- Disappear or alter by four years of age
- Poor prognosis

Myoclonic seizures of childhood

- Occur in children three to twelve years of age
- Characterized by sudden and brief muscular contractions
- May occur in one extremity alone
- Often difficult to control

Akinetic seizures

- Characterized by sudden loss of muscle tone
- Difficult to control

Psychomotor seizures (temporal lobe seizures)

- Characterized by involuntary, repetitive behaviors (e.g., lip smacking, chewing)
- May experience an altered state of consciousness, unusual sensory experiences, or emotional change
- Last from seconds to minutes
- Commonly followed by a state of confusion

Grand mal seizures

- Generalized throughout the body
- May experience a brief warning or aura that can take the form of numbness, noise, taste, smell, or other unusual sensations or feeling
- Tonic phase marked by loss of consciousness, stiffening of the body, irregular breathing, drooling, skin pallor, and incontinence
- Clonic phase is characterized by alternating rigidity and relaxation of the muscles
- Post-ictal phase characterized by drowsiness, disorientation, or fatigue
- Account for approximately 60 percent of all convulsive disorders

Petit mal seizures

- Occur between four and twelve years of age
- Usually disappear at puberty
- One-third to one-half eventually develop grand mal seizures
- Characterized by cessation of activity, staring into space, rapid eye blinking, and a brief loss of consciousness
- No loss of muscle tone
- Brief, usually lasting only 5 to 30 seconds

Focal motor seizures

- Characterized by motor activity
- Restricted to one area
- Caused by abnormal electrical impulse in a localized area of brain
- May become generalized and result in loss of consciousness

Simple febrile seizures

- Most common neurological problems in children under five years of age
- Precipitated by fever
- In infants and children resemble a grand mal seizure
- In neonates characterized by transient reduction in tone or activity; localized motoric movements, twitching of the mouth or face, eye deviations, or an apneic spell
- Usually last less than 5 minutes and seldom longer than 20 minutes

It is estimated that seizure disorders occur in 0.5 percent of the general population (Wolraich, 1984). There are variable causes of seizures, but in many cases, the etiology is unknown. Among known causes are:

- Heredity
- Brain hemorrhage
- Severe head injury
- Hydrocephalus
- Metabolic disorder
- Cerebral palsy
- Myelomeningocele
- Encephalitis
- Meningitis
- Congenital infection

An electroencephalogram (EEG) is usually obtained after behavior characteristic of seizures is noted, to confirm the evidence of a seizure disorder. However, the EEG alone is not sufficient to diagnose a seizure disorder. Seizure disorders may not show up on the EEG; the EEG may be normal despite the fact that behaviors characteristic of seizures are observed, or the EEG pattern may be abnormal even when there is no clinical evidence of seizures. Careful observation of the various clinical manifestations, along with the EEG results, is helpful in confirming a diagnosis. Interventionists should always document and report any suspected seizure activity. Documentation should include:

- Length of seizure
- Description of movement and body parts involved
- Behavior or symptoms just before seizure
- Level of consciousness during and after seizure
- Predisposing factors (illness, fever, etc.)

In many cases anticonvulsant medication can control seizures, once the appropriate dosage requirement has been determined and if the medication is consistently administered. (Wolraich, 1984) (See Table 3).

Table 3
Anticonvulsant Medications and their Side Effects

SEIZURE TYPE	*MEDICATION*	*POSSIBLE SIDE EFFECTS*
Grand mal Focal Psychomotor	Tegretol	Vomiting, drowsiness, headaches, ataxia
Petit mal Myoclonic (Minor motor)	Clonopin	Hyperactivity, dizziness, impulsive behavior, drooling, confusion, drowsiness, ataxia excessive weight gain, short attention span
Infantile Myoclonic	Corticosteroids ACTH	Muscle weakness, Moon face, susceptability to infections, thinning of the bones
Grand mal Psychomotor Focal	Dilantin	Drowsiness, nystagmus, (involuntary, rapid, rhythmic movement of the eyeballs), ataxia, gastric distress)
Grand mal	Phenobarbital	Ataxia, hyperactivity, questionable effect on cognitive performance
Petit mal Grand mal Mixed myoclonic-akinetic	Depakene	Nausea, vomiting, drowsiness

Unfortunately, some children's seizures are not easily controlled and require careful monitoring until the appropriate medication and dosage is determined. Those situations in which seizures may be difficult to control include the following:

- Myoclonic or mixed seizure disorders
- Severe brain injury
- Severe mental retardation

(Wolraich, 1984)

As the child gets older, the seizures may disappear or decrease in frequency, but sometimes one type of seizure is replaced by another (e.g. infantile spasms replaced by grand mal seizures). If the child remains seizure-free for a number of years, the physician will try taking the child off anticonvulsants to see whether seizures will recur.

Neonatal Seizures

Neonates may display different types of seizure characteristics than older children and adults. Seizures in the newborn infant are a significant sign of neurological dysfunction. Seizures in neonates rarely present as classic tonic-clonic (grand mal) seizures; more often, the activity is subtle, characterized by repetitious, non-specific movements. Manifestations of subtle seizures include any of the following:

- Fluttering or blinking of eyelids
- Fixed deviation or rhythmic oscillation of the eyes (nystagmus)
- Drooling
- Mouth movements (e.g. sucking, tongue thrusting, lip smacking)
- Tonic posturing of a limb
- "Bicycling" movement of lower extremities
- Apnea

(Egan & Lierman, 1986)

Interventionists should remember that many neonates display random or abnormal movements. Often these movements are simple jitteriness. Generally, jitteriness subsides when the affected limb is restrained, and is not accompanied by abnormalities of gaze or abnormal eye movement.

Causes of seizures in the neonatal period include:

- Hypoxic-ischemic injury to the brain
- Intracranial hemorrhage
- Metabolic disturbances
- Drug withdrawal
- Central nervous system infection
- Abnormal brain development

If the cause of seizures is unknown, the infant will require diagnostic testing (e.g., EEG, CT Scan, head ultrasonography, lab values) to determine the etiology. Determination of the specific cause of the seizures will assist in planning the most appropriate treatment.

Hydrocephalus

Hydrocephalus is an enlargement of the ventricular system (fluid-filled spaces in and around the brain) from an imbalance in the production and absorption of cerebrospinal fluid in the body. Left untreated, hydrocephalus can cause permanent brain damage.

The primary cause of hydrocephalus is a blockage in the circulation of cerebrospinal fluid. When the normal flow is blocked, the ventricles become filled with this fluid. The blood vessels continue to produce cerebrospinal fluid, and the ventricles begin to enlarge. The enlarging ventricles put pressure on the brain. The increasing fluid causes the infant's head to enlarge and the soft spots (fontanelles) to bulge. As the child grows older and the fontanelles close, the head will no longer be able to accommodate the fluid build-up. Left untreated, hydrocephalus can result in brain damage.

Two types of blockages exist:

1. **Noncommunicating hydrocephalus** - results when the outflow of cerebrospinal fluid from the ventricles is blocked.
2. **Communicating hydrocephalus** - results when the cerebrospinal fluid passes out of the ventricles but is blocked from being re-absorbed.

The signs and symptoms of an infant with hydrocephalus include:

- Increased head circumference
- Dilated scalp veins
- Bulging fontanelles
- Separation of cranial suture lines
- Setting sun sign of the eye (downward gaze of eyes so that the white area above the pupil is prominent)
- Listlessness
- Shrill and high-pitched cry
- Irritability
- Vomiting
- Developmental delays

In older children, whose skulls can no longer expand, the symptoms of hydrocephalus are more acute; they include:

- Headache
- Vomiting
- Coma

When hydrocephalus is suspected, a specialized X-ray (CAT scan, MRI, or ultrasound in infants) may be performed to observe the structure of the brain and determine if the ventricles are dilated, thereby confirming the diagnosis of hydrocephalus.

With proper medical and neurosurgical management, the majority of children with hydrocephalus will survive, although 60 percent will have significant intellectual and motor disabilities (Wolraich, 1984).

The neurosurgical goal for the infant with hydrocephalus is to decrease the amount of pressure building up within the brain by the removal of the obstruction or, if this is not possible, diversion of the CSF from the ventricles into another body cavity. If the cause of the hydrocephalus is an overproduction of cerebrospinal fluid, medication may be used to reduce the amount of CSF produced. The most commonly used treatment involves the surgical placement of a shunt. Shunts divert the CSF from the ventricles, either to the peritoneal cavity (ventriculoperitoneal shunt) or to the atrial cavity of the heart (ventriculoatrial shunt). In infants, the placement of a ventriculoperitoneal (VP) shunt is often the method of choice. An extra length of catheter is generally coiled in the peritoneum to extend as the infant grows.

Interventionists working with children who have shunts should be aware of the signs of shunt failure and infection, the two major potential complications related to shunts. The symptoms of shunt obstruction in infants are identical to the signs and symptoms of hydrocephalus as previously noted.

Infection of the shunt can result in ventriculitis (inflammation of the ventricles) or meningitis (inflammation of the membranes covering the brain and spinal cord). The infant may show signs of shunt obstruction. Fever, redness, tenderness or puffiness along the shunt tract may be noted. Abdominal distension and tenderness may also be indications of shunt infection.

The long-range prognosis for infants with hydrocephalus depends on the cause and severity of the hydrocephalus and the effectiveness of treatment. Repeated hospitalizations for shunt revisions and treatment of infection are common occurrences for children with shunts.

While many children with hydrocephalus have no specific educational problems, others may sustain damage to the brain which results in motor, language, perceptual or intellectual disabilities. Rote memory characteristically is a relative strength for these children, and their verbal skills sometimes make them appear more able than they are overall (Wolraich, 1984).

Cerebral Palsy

Cerebral palsy (CP) is a term that refers to a variety of nonprogressive neurologic disabilities caused by injuries in the prenatal or perinatal period. These injuries to the central nervous system result in abnormalities of motor functioning. Because the definition of CP is not very precise, exact statistics are unavailable. It is estimated that the incidence of cerebral palsy is about 7 in 1000 live births and the prevalence is about 500 cases per 100,000 population. Children with CP may have normal intelligence, although it has been estimated that significant cognitive delays are present in 30 percent to 70 percent of children with CP (Behrman & Kliegman, 1990). The causes of CP include the following:

- Developmental anomalies
- Congenital infection
- Perinatal trauma
- Metabolic disorders in the perinatal period

A wide range of neuromotor dysfunctions exist in children with cerebral palsy, depending upon the area of the brain involved. Cerebral palsy is classified into several distinct patterns, which are described below by Behrman & Kliegman (1990):

<u>Spastic diplegia</u>

- Occurs most frequently in low birthweight.
- Is associated with birth asphyxia or intraventricular hemorrhage.
- Involves the lower extremities more than the upper.
- Is characterized by increased muscle tone (spasticity), increased deep tendon reflexes, and a Babinsky reflex in the legs.
- Severe mental retardation is less common than in other forms of CP.
- Hip, knee, and ankle contractures interfere with ambulation.

<u>Spastic quadriplegia</u>

- Involves all four extremities.
- Is associated with low birthweight and severe birth asphyxia.
- Is often seen in conjunction with mental retardation, seizures, and feeding difficulties.

<u>Spastic hemiplegia</u>

- Is associated with injury to one brain hemisphere.

- Motor deficits are seen on the opposite side of the body from the brain lesion.
- Cognitive deficits relate to those functions of the side of the brain that is involved.

Extrapyramidal CP

- Is characterized by hypotonia, choreoathetosis, and dystonic movements.
- Is most often associated with the highly elevated newborn bilirubin levels (kernicterus) .
- Cognitive function is more often normal than in other forms of CP.
- Hearing impairment is common.

Atonic CP

- Is associated with marked hypotonia.
- Brisk reflexes.
- Severe cognitive delays.

Mixed forms

- Due to combinations of insults to multiple cerebral areas.
- Typically associated with sensory deficits, seizures, and cognitive/perceptual impairments.

The primary treatment of CP is through physical and occupational therapies to enhance movement and increase function of the affected parts of the body. Surgical intervention may be necessary to correct orthopedic problems, such as tight tendons and joint contractures. Medications such as Valium may be helpful to relax muscles.

Myelomeningocele

Myelomeningocele, or Spina Bifida, is a defect of the skin, spinal column and spinal cord. It involves the incomplete fusion of the vertebrae during the first trimester of pregnancy, resulting in the improper formation of the spinal cord. Normally, the meninges (membranes surrounding the spinal cord) and the spinal cord containing the nerves are protected within the spinal column. In the infant with myelomeningocele, a particular section of vertebrae along the spinal column does not fuse properly during fetal development. As a result, the meninges pouch out at the break along the spinal column and form a sack. As the spinal cord develops down the spinal column, it follows out the break and enters the sack. (See Figure A.)

Myelomeningocele is just one type of spinal defect; two others are:

- Meningocele - The meninges form the sack, but the spinal cord remains within the vertebrae.
- Spina bifida occulta - The vertebrae dos not completely fuse, but there are no abnormalities in the meninges, spinal cord or skin.

The initial diagnosis of myelomeningocele may be made prior to birth by ultrasound or amniocentesis, or at the time of birth by physical examination. In rare cases, the defect can go undetected in the newborn period because it is covered by skin.

The location of the defect may occur anywhere along the spinal column. The higher up the defect is on the spinal column, the greater the neuromuscular involvement. Most of the defects are located in the thoracic, lumbar, or sacral regions of the

Figure A

Spinal Cord Defects (Whaley & Wong, 1991 by Permission)

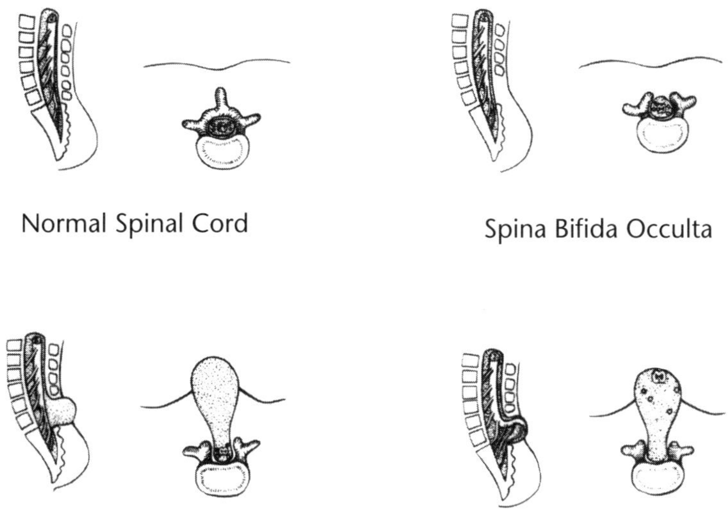

spine (Wolraich, 1984). The long-term effects are determined by the location of the defect and the degree of neural involvement. Thus, an infant with a myelomeningocele located above the twelfth thoracic vertebrae will have no voluntary leg movement. An infant with a spina bifida occulta defect at the fifth lumbar vertebrae will usually have little or no neuromuscular impairment. Additional health problems are often associated with myelomeningocele. They include:

- Hydrocephalus
- Bladder and bowel problems (neurogenic bladder, constipation and incontinence)
- Curvature of the spine (scoliosis)
- Pressure sores (decubitus ulcers)

To prevent infections to the spinal area and brain, surgical intervention is usually performed within the first 24 to 48 hours after birth to close the back lesion. Another surgical procedure is usually performed within the first few months of life to place a shunt to reduce the effects of hydrocephalus.

Interventionists working with children who have shunts should monitor the children for signs of either shunt malfunction or infection (see hydrocephalus). In addition, interventionists should note any sign of pressure sores. Many children with myelomeningocele are somewhat immobile and lack sensation in their lower extremities, making them prone to pressure sores. Pressure sores result from the skin breaking down and can lead to severe infection. Redness of the skin is the first sign of problems. Strategies to prevent skin breakdown are as follows:

- Reposition the child frequently
- Allow for good circulation; avoid tight clothing
- Keep the child off toys or small sharp objects
- Keep skin clean and dry. (This may be difficult due to lack of bowel and bladder control)
- Inspect skin frequently

Many children with myelomeningocele are also prone to urinary tract infections due to neurogenic bladders. Neurogenic bladder refers to a child's inability to feel the urge to urinate or a lack of control of the urinary sphincter. If not cared for properly, a neurogenic bladder can lead to urine retention within the bladder, which in turn can lead to urinary tract infection and subsequent kidney damage. A bladder regime involving catheterization and periodic assessment of urinary tract function helps prevent urinary tract infection. Interventionists should note and report any of the signs and symptoms of a urinary tract infection. A simple urine test can be obtained to verify any suspicions. Symptoms of urinary tract infection in an infant include:

- Unexplained fever
- Colic
- Abdominal distress
- Anorexia
- Vomiting
- Jaundice
- Blood in the urine

The extent of physical and intellectual problems associated with myelomeningocele vary with the location of the defect. Children with accompanying hydrocephalus are at greater risk for developing learning disabilities and mental retardation. The constant occurrence of acute problems such as shunt malfunctions, urinary tract infection, and repeated hospitalizations and surgery also place a child at risk for developmental delays (Wolraich, 1984).

KIDNEY DYSFUNCTION

One of the primary functions of the kidneys is to filter out the waste products from the blood and to excrete these waste products in the form of urine. This process maintains an appropriate chemical balance of body fluids; in contrast, kidney (or renal) dysfunction or failure is an inability of the kidneys to maintain the normal chemical balance. Three types of disorders exist:

- Acute kidney failure
- Chronic kidney failure
- End-stage kidney failure

Acute kidney failure, uncommon in childhood, is characterized by a sudden and often short-term failure of the kidneys to regulate appropriately the volume and composition of urine. Chronic kidney failure commences when diseased or damaged kidneys can no longer maintain the normal chemical composition of body fluids under normal conditions. It is characterized by a progressive deterioration over a period of time which produces a variety of clinical and biochemical disturbances and eventually leads to end-stage failure. End-stage kidney failure is the most severe of the three disorders and is considered terminal without dialysis or transplantation (Whaley & Wong, 1991). For the purpose of this discussion, we will focus on chronic and end-stage failure.

A variety of diseases and disorders can cause chronic renal failure in young children. The most frequent causes of chronic renal failure in infants and young children (under age five) are:

- Congenital kidney malformation
- Congenital urinary tract malformation
- Vesicoureteral reflux (reflux of bladder urine into the ureters)

(Whaley & Wong, 1991)

The diagnosis of chronic renal failure is usually made on the basis of clinical signs and symptoms, medical history prior to kidney disease, and on biochemical findings. The onset is usually gradual, and the initial signs and symptoms are vague and nonspecific. As the kidneys continue to deteriorate, the clinical signs and symptoms of the kidney dysfunction become more apparent. There symptoms frequently include:

- Growth failure
- Weight loss
- Anemia
- Malaise
- Pallor
- Facial puffiness
- Bone or joint pain
- Increased urination
- Headache
- Muscle cramps
- Dry or itchy skin
- Bruised skin

Children with chronic renal failure are particularly susceptible to infections, especially pneumonia and urinary tract infections. In addition, these children frequently are hypertensive (high blood pressure) and usually demonstrate neurologic manifestations as the disease process progresses.

The medical management of chronic renal failure varies according to the progression of the disease but the basic goals are to:

- Promote effective renal function.
- Maintain body fluid and electrolyte balance.
- Treat systemic complications.
- Promote a normal and active life for as long as possible.

At some point in the disease process—typically shortly before end-stage failure, the physician must either place the child on kidney dialysis or perform a kidney transplant.

A kidney transplant is the treatment of choice in the pediatric age group because it leads to improved body growth and offers a greater chance for a normal lifestyle. It is also less expensive than a chronic dialysis program (Elias & Bauer, 1989). Indeed, most children respond favorably to kidney transplant, with the majority returning to a relatively normal life within a year after such surgery (Whaley & Wong, 1991).

Often children with chronic kidney failure will have to undergo dialysis, even if for a short time prior to transplantation surgery. Interventionists should be aware of the two methods of dialysis currently available for the management of renal failure:

1. **Peritoneal dialysis** - also known as continuous ambulatory peritoneal dialysis, (CAPD) is the dialysis of choice for small infants because no vascular access is necessary (Elias & Bauer, 1989). In peritoneal dialysis, the membranes within the abdominal cavity, together with a special dialysis fluid, filter out the impurities from the body. To gain access to the abdominal cavity, a catheter is surgically inserted into the abdomen. The dialysis solution is then allowed to flow into the abdominal cavity where it remains while the waste products seep from the abdomen into the fluid. The fluid is then drained by gravity. This painless procedure is repeated on a daily basis for as long as possible. One advantage of this type of dialysis is that it can be performed at home by a trained family member. Inflammation of the abdominal cavity (peritonitis) is a major complication associated with this type of dialysis and requires prompt medical attention.

   Signs and symptoms of peritonitis include:
   - Vomiting
   - Progressive abdominal distention
   - Increased heart rate
   - Rapid shallow breathing
   - Irritability
   - Pallor
   - Chills
   - Restlessness
   - A characteristic side-lying position with the knees flexed to the abdomen

2. **Hemodialysis** purifies the blood through the use of a specialized piece of equipment called a hemodialyzer or artificial kidney. The blood is circulated outside the body through this artificial kidney and then returned to the body. In order to gain access to the blood, a surgical procedure is performed to create an external or internal arterioveneous shunt, usually in the arm. Two needles must be inserted into the shunt site each time the child requires hemodialysis—usually two or three times per week. These shunt sites are prone to infections and clogging. Children on dialysis must follow a strict diet to restrict excess salt and fluid. Most children show rapid improvement in their growth rate and skeletal maturation with the implementation of dialysis, although they rarely achieve a normal growth pattern. Seizures are a common side effect of hemodialysis. As with CAPD, hemodialysis can be done at home following the proper training and education of the parent (Whaley & Wong, 1991).

Chronic kidney failure must be treated with drugs and artificial filtering; as a result, many stresses are placed on these children and their families. Moreover, the progressive deterioration of kidney functioning is irreversible, and both the child and family must accept the disheartening prospect of dependence on dialysis or a transplant. As the child with kidney disease progresses from kidney insufficiency to end-stage kidney failure and then to hemodialysis and transplantation, the need for supportive care is intensified (Whaley & Wong, 1991).

ACQUIRED IMMUNE DEFICIENCY SYNDROME (AIDS)

A relatively new condition is the subject of much discussion as to appropriate management within early intervention programs: Acquired Immune Deficiency Syndrome (AIDS).

AIDS is a disease in which the human immunodeficiency virus (HIV) infects and impairs certain immune cells of the body, leaving the body vulnerable to infections and cancerous growths. The diagnosis of "full-blown" or "true" AIDS is made when manifestations of such opportunistic infections and cancerous growths appear. Prior to the onset of full-blown AIDS, a person may have some symptoms related to HIV infection, but not true AIDS; these persons are classified as having AIDS-related complex. There are also many persons who exhibit no symptoms of the disease but test seropositive for the antibodies of the virus; these persons are known to be "HIV positive." These individuals can transmit the virus even though they may have no symptoms.

The human immunodeficiency virus is transmitted among humans by either sexual contact or the infusion of infected blood from another person. With respect to infants, HIV infection is generally acquired through blood products or by transmission from the mother during pregnancy and delivery. With improved screening of blood products, the number of new children infected with the virus via blood transfusion should become virtually nonexistent in the next decade. In contrast, due to the increasing number of HIV-infected women of childbearing age, the number of children born to HIV-infected mothers is likely to increase substantially in the coming years (Anderson, 1988).

Anderson (1988) describes three possible outcomes that are likely when an HIV-infected woman gives birth:

1. A small percentage of the newborns, having become infected in utero with the human immunodeficiency virus, will exhibit the clinical features of congenital HIV syndrome. These babies will suffer from growth failure, respiratory infections, and neurological involvement and will therefore require early intervention services.
2. In 30 percent to 50 percent of cases, the newborn will appear normal at the time of birth, but will become symptomatic early in life.
3. About 50 percent of infants will not become infected despite their mothers HIV+ status.

Antibody levels in newborns, the key indicator of infection, are difficult to interpret during the first year of life because the infant will show evidence of maternal antibodies that have passed across the placenta. While it should be presumed initially that all newborns of HIV-infected mothers are HIV-infected themselves, only if the HIV antibodies persist beyond the first twelve to fifteen months of life is it believed to reflect a true HIV infection of the infant.

In contrast to adults who may remain symptom-free for ten years after infection, children infected at birth with the human immunovirus usually become symptomatic at a relatively early stage in life (Anderson, 1988).

The clinical signs and symptoms of an infant with active HIV-infection include:

- Weight loss
- Diarrhea
- Failure to thrive
- Diaphoresis (profuse sweating)

- Chronic cough
- Developmental delays
- Neurologic deficits
- Microcephaly
- Frequent ear and/or respiratory infections
- Oral thrush

(Berry, 1988)

The medical goal for these children includes keeping them well nourished and protected from opportunistic infection. Because these children have compromised immune systems, ordinary infections may become life-threatening. Interventionists must be particularly careful to protect these infants from infections during their therapy sessions. Therefore, it is very important for interventionists to be aware of and to practice appropriate infection control. A few simple steps taken throughout the day can help prevent the spread of infection:

- Wash hands frequently after handling another child
- Wash toys and equipment with a 1:10 mixture of chlorine bleach and water after using with another child
- Avoid working with children if you yourself have a viral infection that day

These steps should be taken with all children, not just children who are HIV-infected. Most children with chronic illnesses are at risk for developing infections, and these simple steps will help reduce such risk.

One concern frequently discussed among interventionists is the risk of infection to themselves. Studies continue to show that the risk of HIV transmission among health care workers (as well as family members) is exceedingly low. The few cases where transmission to health care workers has occurred have involved unusual circumstances with exposure to substantial quantities of blood (Anderson, 1988). This does not mean that interventionists should be cavalier when handling body secretions of children. The risk of contracting hepatitis B in particular remains significant and should be reason enough to practice stringent hygenic techniques. Therefore, the following universal precautions should be utilized with all children:

- Wear gloves when changing diapers or cleaning up blood spills
- Wash hands immediately following exposure to bodily secretion or fluids

Finally, children who are HIV-infected require the same amount of love and emotional support that all children need. Remember that children with AIDS present no risk in being touched, hugged, and loved.

Interacting with Medical Professionals and Medical Technology

Early Interventionists who work with developmentally delayed children with chronic illnesses should be cognizant of the general characteristics of their child's health problems and the limitations such problems place on the child. In addition, these illnesses will require early interventionists to interact, to one degree or another, with medical professionals and with sophisticated medical technology. How should the interventionist approach these aspects of the child's care routine?

With respect to medical technology, an early interventionist may come into contact with a variety of equipment in both the home and hospital settings, including oxygen saturation monitors, apnea monitors, suction machines, ventilators, and hemodialyzers. It is well beyond the scope of this chapter to provide a thorough grounding in the mechanical functions of such equipment. Indeed, interventionists are rarely responsible for the day-to-day operation and maintenance of such equipment. The degree of competence necessary to operate and maintain such equipment is obtained only through many hours of training and experience. Interventionists who are engaged to work with a child dependent on medical technology should not operate machinery independently, and they should not go beyond their area of responsibility, lest they put the child at medical risk. On the other hand, interventionists should be familiar with the child's medical condition. The interventionist should consult closely with the child's caregiver and physician to understand the child's limitations. The interventionists should learn the physical indicators that signal distress in the event that medical assistance must be summoned.

To provide optimal care for the child, effective communication among the interventionists, parents, and the medical professionals who are providing care for the child is essential. Such communication is not always easy to facilitate, in part because of the large number of medical professionals involved in the care of a chronically ill child. For example, children suffering from a cardiac defect may receive outpatient care from the following:

- Pediatric cardiovascular surgeon
- Pediatric cardiologist
- Primary pediatrician
- Cardiac nurse practitioner
- Social worker
- Nutritionist
- Visiting nurse or home-based nurse

Interventionists can enhance the likelihood of effective communication by maintaining regular contacts with the doctors and other medical professionals caring for the child. With the parents' permission, interventionists should initiate the following contacts:

- Visiting the physician with the child and parent
- Phoning the physician with questions or concerns about the child's condition
- Inviting the physician to consultative sessions involving the child's developmental plan
- Providing written developmental summaries, IFSP's and regular progress reports to the physician

Many chronically ill children must remain hospitalized for significant periods. In such cases, it is important for interventionists to maintain communication with the child's hospital caregivers. Interventionists should ascertain the identities of all the medical professionals involved in the child's care to best assure that the child's developmental goals become a part of the medical management plan. To use the same example of the child with a cardiac defect, the following professionals may be involved during the child's hospitalization:

- Attending physician (intensivist)
- Resident physician (house staff)
- Cardiologist
- Floor nurses (rotating by shift)
- Primary nurse
- Child-life staff

- Nutritionist
- Social worker

Regular consultation with the child's primary care nurse is essential for implementation of the child's medical and developmental plan during hospitalization. While telephone contacts are useful for periodic update, direct contact with the child, parents and medical professionals remains important.

REFERENCES

Ahmann, E. (1986). *Home care for the high risk infant: A holistic guide to using technology.* Rockville, MD: Aspen Publications.

Anderson, R.D. (1988). Management of developmentally disabled children with chronic infections. *Infants and Young Children, 1*(1),1-9.

Behrman, R.E. & Kliegman, R. (1990). *Nelson essentials of pediatrics.* Philadelphia: W.B. Saunders.

Berry, R.K. (1988). Home care of the child with AIDS. *Pediatric Nursing, 12*(4), 341-344.

Blackman, J.A. (1984). *Medical aspects of developmental disabilities in children birth to three.* Rockville, MD: Aspen Publications.

Bozynski, M.E.A. (1989). Comprehensive management of the infant with bronchopulmonary dysplasia: A growing challenge. *Infants and Young Children, 2*(1), 14-24.

Egan, J.O. & Lierman, C. J. (1986). Home care of the infant with seizures. In E. Ahmann (Ed.), *Home care for the high risk infant: A holistic guide to using technology* (pp. 225-245). Rockville, MD: Aspen Publications.

Elias, E.R. & Bauer, S.B. (1989). Urologic disorders. In I.L. Rubin & A.C. Crocker (Eds.), *Developmental disabilities: Delivery of medical care for children and adults* (pp. 282-303). Philadelphia: Lea and Febiger.

Ensher, G.L. & Clark, D.A. (1986). *Newborns at risk: Medical care and psychoeducational intervention.* Rockville, MD: Aspen Publications.

Gantt, L. & Thompson, C. (1985). Short gut syndrome in the infant. *American Journal of Nursing,* 85(11), 1263-1266.

Harrison, H. (1983). *The premature baby book: A parents' guide to coping and caring in the first year.* New York: St. Martins' Press.

Higgins, S.S. (1987). Patterns of impairment: Congenital heart defects. In M.H. Rose & R.B. Thomas (Eds.), *Children with chronic conditions: Nursing in a family and community context* (pp. 165-185). Orlando, FL: Grune and Stratton Inc.

Hobbs, N., Perrin, J.M., & Ireys, H.T. (1985). *Chronically ill children and their families: Problems, prospects, and proposals from the Vanderbilt study.* San Francisco: Jossey-Bass Publishers.

Ichord, R. (1986). Profile of the high risk infant. In E. Ahmann (Ed.), *Home care for the high risk infant: A holistic guide to using technology* (pp. 1-11). Rockville, MD: Aspen Publications.

Pettett, G. (1986). Medical complications of the premature infant. In J.K. Sweeney

(Ed.), *The high risk neonates: Developmental therapy perspectives* (pp. 91-104). New York: Haworth Press.

Simon, B.M. (1986). Speech and language development in the high risk infant. In E. Ahmann (Ed.), *Home care for the high risk infant: A holistic guide to using technology* (pp. 261-270). Rockville, MD: Aspen Publications.

Vaucher, Y.E. (1988). Understanding intraventricular hemorrhage and white-matter injury in premature infants. *Infants and Young Children 1*(2), 31-45.

Whaley, L.F. & Wong, D.L. (1991). *Nursing care of infants and children.* 4th Edition. St. Louis, MO: Mosby - Year Book, Inc.

Wolraich, M.L. (1984). Hydrocephalus. In J.A. Blackman (Ed.), *Medical aspects of developmental disabilities in children birth to three* (pp. 137-141). Rockville, MD: Aspen Publications.

Wolraich, M.L. (1984). Myelomeningocele. In J.A. Blackman (Ed.), *Medical aspects of developmental disabilities in children birth to three* (pp. 159-165). Rockville, MD: Aspen Publications.

Wolraich, M.L. (1984). Seizure disorders. In J.A. Blackman (Ed.), *Medical aspects of developmental disabilities in children birth to three* (pp. 215-221). Rockville, MD: Aspen Publications.

Chapter 3

Project Headed Home: A Model for Serving Hospitalized Infants and their Families

Kathy S. Katz, Ph.D.

The increased survival of chronically ill children results in more of them being discharged from hospitals to home care. Due to their fragile medical status, however, these children are often back in the hospital as they cope with acute illness or setbacks caused by their chronic conditions. Some of these hospital stays are brief, lasting only for a few days. At other times, a child must remain in the hospital many months until her condition is stable enough once again to return home. For their families, these rehospitalizations upset the delicate balance they maintain when the child is able to be cared for at home. The families may require a variety of support services to help them cope with the stress that a hospitalization understandably causes. While a child's medical needs during hospitalization are paramount, her emotional and educational needs must be addressed to maintain her psychological health during and after hospitalization.

The chronically ill child becomes well known to the personnel at the hospital. Certain staff members will often form close personal relationships with the child and his family through their frequent or prolonged contact. They can be a great support to the child and his family by providing continuity in services. Because they know the family, staff members are able to adapt routines to fit the particular needs of a family.

Medical care providers in hospitals (physicians, nurses and therapists) are often interested in knowing what strategies they might apply to better meet the many needs of the chronically ill infant and her family. Guidelines for service delivery and specific techniques to use with this population have emerged from recent investigations of exemplary service provision for these infants.

Project Headed Home of the Georgetown University Hospital Child Development Center was developed as an early intervention program specifically for chronically ill infants and their families. The program was designed to provide direct service during the child's hospitalization in the Pediatric Intensive Care Unit (PICU)) and to assist the family in transition to home care. The project was funded by a Handicapped

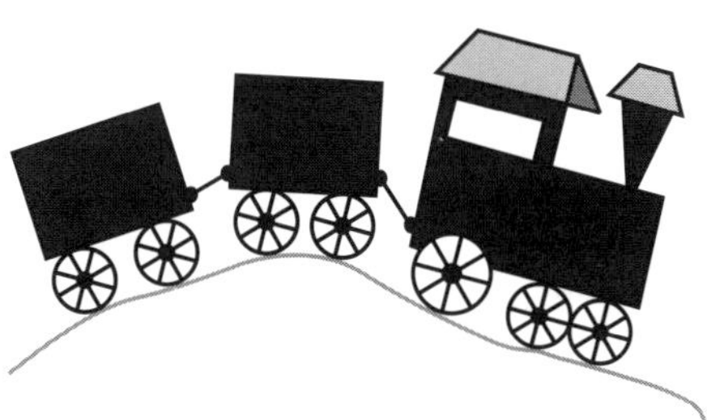

Children's Early Education Program Grant through the U.S. Department of Education, Office of Special Education Programs. This funding program supports the refinement of models for exemplary service delivery to children with disabilities.

PROJECT HEADED HOME

Project Headed Home was designed to serve chronically ill and medically fragile infants and their families who, because of prolonged or frequent hospitalizations in the PICU, are unable to participate in community-based early intervention programs. Intervention is provided during the PICU stay through direct service to the infant, training and social support to the parents, and suggestions to medical and nursing caregivers concerning developmental needs of the child.

A diagram of the project scheme appears in Figure B.

Figure B
Project Headed Home
Diagrammatic Scheme

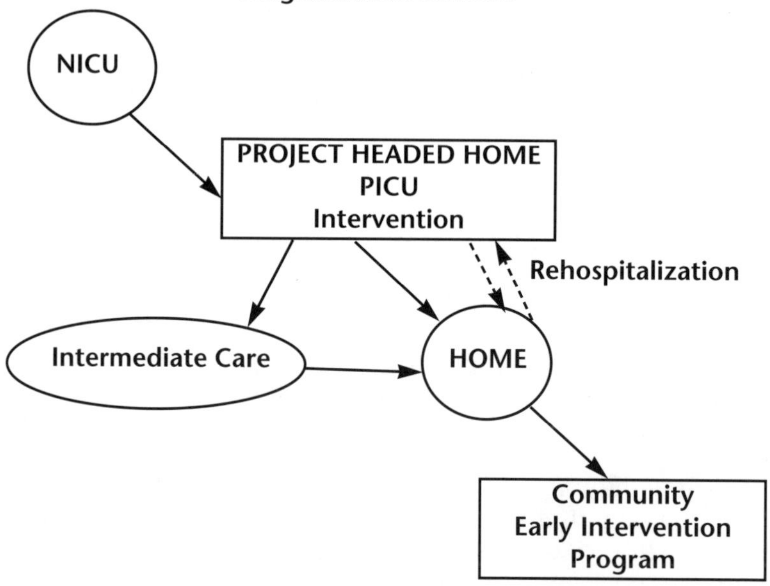

Headed Home originated at a time when far-reaching federal legislation was being enacted that would expand eligibility for infants with disabilities for early intervention services. The legislation incorporated some of the philosophical changes described previously regarding the role of the family of the infant in respect to intervention. The new legislation, IDEA Part H, shifted the focus of the intervention from the child alone toward the needs of the family as a whole.

This shift to family-centered intervention is an integral part of the philosophy and application of the Headed Home goals. Family-centered care includes identifying and responding to the needs of the total family and collaborating with the family in all phases of service delivery. In Project Headed Home, professionals and families work together to balance the professional recommendations with the priorities of the families so the strategies that are developed truly reflect family needs or goals.

TARGET POPULATION

The chronically ill infants and their families appropriate for the Headed Home intervention model present a broad range of medical conditions. The common feature is the need for ongoing medical caregiving in the home, frequently depending on medical technological supports, and the likelihood of repeated hospitalization. Guidelines of typical medical complications that would lead to the child's being considered appropriate for the intervention model include the following:

- Infants with continuing needs for hospitalization transferring from the Neonatal Intensive Care Unit to the Pediatric Intensive Care Unit
- Infants with chronic bronchopulmonary dysplasia resulting in frequent, severe respiratory infections
- Extremely low birthweight prematures less than 1000 grams
- Infants with congenital abnormalities who require repeated hospitalizations
- Infants with central nervous system impairment who require ongoing medical management
- Infants with chronic renal failure
- Failure-to-thrive infants

This list is certainly not exhaustive. Family social issues that might make it difficult for a particular family to manage their child's medical condition at home also represent a risk situation appropriate for the model.

IDENTIFICATION PROCEDURES

Children meeting the above criteria are identified through a variety of channels. Participation by a member of the Headed Home team in the weekly **social service rounds** for the inpatient services is the most common route. At this meeting, attended by the nurse coordinator, social worker, child-life staff, attending physician or resident, psychologist and Headed Home team member, each of the inpatient children is discussed in regards to addressing family needs. If the child fits the guidelines for enrollment, the Headed Home staff member requests a physician's approval to approach the family about participation.

Other referrals come **directly from the nursing staff** on the inpatient services. The nursing staff, which experiences a substantial yearly turnover, is kept aware of the project through a variety of strategies, including:

- A supply of Headed Home brochures kept at the nurses' station
- Workshop sessions by Headed Home staff as part of the nursing in-service series
- A changing bulletin board on the ward highlighting aspects of inpatient early intervention
- Direct contact with Headed Home team members, who provide consultation to the nursing staff about already enrolled infants.

Once the child's physician has given approval, one member of the Headed Home team is designated to be the service coordinator and to meet with the family to explain the project to them. The role of the service coordinator is an extremely important one and will be described in detail in the following section.

TEAM CONSTELLATION

The Project Headed Home team was designed to be an interdisciplinary one. Specific role definitions were formulated for a member from a particular discipline. The roles are intended to be complementary, but in a number of instances, several team members are able to fulfill a similar role. Thus, the functional roles of the team are both interdisciplinary and transdisciplinary.

The Headed Home team is composed of:

- A psychologist
- An infant specialist
- A pediatric physical therapist
- A speech-language pathologist
- A nurse specialist

A diagram of the team organization appears in Figure C. Each team member participates in the assessment process for the infant and family at the time of initial enrollment, and each is involved in the formulation of the intervention plan. Direct

Figure C
Project Headed Home
Team Organization

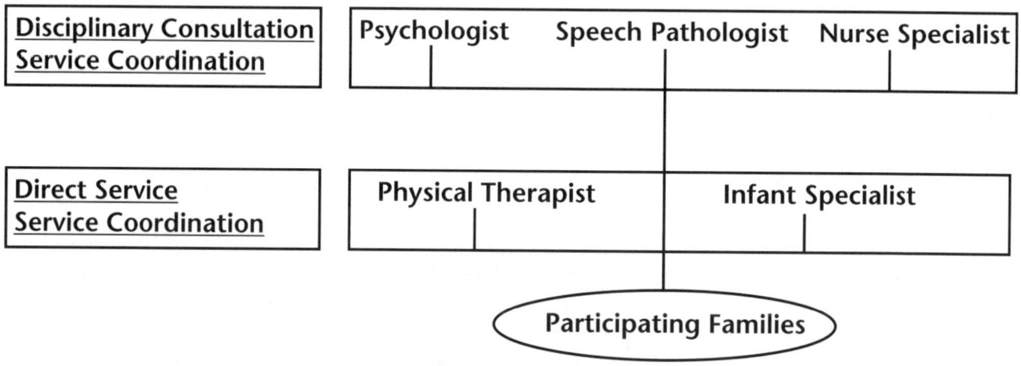

service to the infant and consultation to the parent and medical staff are done primarily by the **infant specialist** and **physical therapist**. Other team members provide independent consultation to the family or medical caregivers as needed, but they provide regular input to the Project Headed Home team in program planning for each participating infant and family. Each member of the team serves as a service coordinator for several families. Activities associated with the function of a team member of a specific discipline are outlined in Table 4.

These roles were developed to use disciplinary expertise to the full advantage. Service coordination responsibility and direct service delivery, on the other hand, often involve transdisciplinary functioning. This means that the infant specialist may work with the family on motor goals recommended by the physical therapist, or the physical therapist may provide family support as suggested through consultation with the psychologist. This is an important concept in that it may make service provision more efficient and more integrated. Transdisciplinary function may also reduce stress on the family by reducing the number of professionals with whom they need to interact.

Table 4
Project Headed Home
Roles and Responsibilities of Team Members

INFANT SPECIALIST

* Serves as liaison with PICU nursing administration
* Coordinates daily project activities
* Assists in identifying infants for enrollment
* Provides service coordination
* Provides family support as needed
* Assists in recommending developmental objectives for the infant and family
* Provides developmental intervention to infants
* Communicates with PICU staff and family on providing activities to meet developmental goals
* Assists in identifying post-discharge needs and community resources for meeting needs
* Assists in preparing community-based intervention agencies to meet needs of infant and family

PEDIATRIC PHYSICAL THERAPIST

* Provides service coordination
* Provides family support as needed
* Performs neuromotor assessment on enrolled infants
* Assists in recommending neuromotor objectives for infant and family
* Provides neuromotor intervention to the infant as needed, including use of appropriate adaptive equipment
* Communicates with PICU staff and family in providing activities to meet neuromotor goals as needed
* Assists in identifying post-discharge motor needs and appropriate community resources for meeting those needs

NURSE SPECIALIST

* Provides service coordination
* Consults with team regarding implications of medical condition on the developmental plan
* Assists in identifying family needs around medical caregiving
* Assists in providing parent training in medical management
* Assists in identifying post-discharge medical needs and appropriate community resources for meeting those needs
* Assists family in their transition to home management of medical and developmental needs
* Assists in coordination of home health care plan
* Provides information and any needed guidance around health needs to community-based intervention program enrolling child

Table 4 (continued)

PSYCHOLOGIST

* Provides overall direction, implementation, and evaluation of the project
* Assists in identifying infants for enrollment
* Provides service coordination
* Provides consultation to the team in regards to enhancing parent-developmental team PICU staff-developmental team, and the child-interventionist collaborations
* Assists service coordinator in family needs assessment formulations
* Provides assessment of child's cognitive and social adaptive level
* Assists in recommending cognitive and behavioral objectives for the infant and family
* Provides supportive short-term counseling or behavior management counseling to families as needed
* Assists in identifying post-discharge developmental needs for infant and family and appropriate community resources to meet them

SPEECH-LANGUAGE PATHOLOGIST

* Provides service coordination
* Performs assessment of child's oral-motor function, feeding skills, speech and language, and interpersonal communication skills, as needed
* Assists in recommending objectives in regards to the above for the child and his family
* Provides consultation and modeling to the team, parents and PICU staff of the intervention strategies to achieve the objectives
* Assists in identifying post-discharge needs for the above areas of function and community resources available to meet them
* Provides consultation to community-based resources serving the infant as to strategies to meet developmental objectives, as needed

PROJECT GOALS

Project Headed Home was designed to influence the caregiving techniques of those people in the chronically ill infant's life who would have the greatest potential for implementing a developmental plan. The Headed Home team directs activities to three major target groups with different goals designated for each group. The three target groups include:

1. The family of the hospitalized child
2. The chronically ill infant
3. Medical/nursing caregiving staff

Project goals for enhancing the **Family** capability for intervening with the child include:

- Development of a collaborative relationship with medical caregivers and developmental team
- Determination of resources and needs of the parents themselves and their child
- Development of competence in the management of their child's medical and developmental needs

- Incorporation of developmental activities into caregiving routines in the hospital and at home
- Developing awareness of community resources and advocating needed services for their child

Specific goals for the **Infant** to be achieved by the intervention program include:

- Development of more mature state regulation and autonomic control
- Medical stability
- Normalized routines in the hospital and at home
- Enhancement of development in areas of cognitive, motor, language, and psychosocial functioning

To accomplish the foregoing child and family goals, a close working relationship among family, project staff and pediatric intensive care staff is essential. To ensure the integration of developmental and medical needs into the caregiving plan, goals are directed to **medical/nursing staff**, as follows:

- The ability to select toys and activities appropriate to the developmental level of each child
- Knowledge of the implications of specific medical conditions on a child's risk for developmental problems
- Understanding normal developmental expectations so that infants showing delay can be brought to the attention of developmental staff

PICU staff must take two major avenues to achieve these goals. The first is through direct consultation about the needs of individual infants. The second is through specific presentations and workshops incorporated into the nurses' ongoing in-service series. Prior to development of the in-service sessions, nurses were surveyed to ascertain what specific questions they had in regards to development in chronically ill infants. They identified the following areas of concern which they felt represented the greatest need for information:

- Communicating with hospitalized infants, toddlers, and their families to maintain a family-centered approach
- Interventions for enhancing neuromotor development of hospitalized infants (positioning, handling, and adaptive equipment)
- Effects of the hospital environment on infants, toddlers, and their families

PROJECT ACTIVITIES

ENROLLMENT

When an infant is identified as appropriate for the project, a service coordinator, who may be any member of the team, is assigned to the family. After obtaining consent for participation from the family, the service coordinator begins the process of assessing the infant's and family's resources and needs.

The Assessment Process

The service coordinator meets with the parents to discuss their observations of the child's functioning and their goals for her development and also to explore the needs of the family as a whole. The service coordinator shares this information at a weekly Headed Home team meeting to elicit suggestions for assessment strategies. These recommendations are then discussed with the family, and an assessment plan is agreed upon.

The part of the assessment plan focusing on the **infant** usually includes objective measures of *cognitive, language, and neuromotor functioning*. Assessment of *feeding skills* is also often a part, in that the nutritional status of chronically ill children is frequently a concern. *Social interactive skills* are observed during caregiving by parents and hospital staff. Observations by the nursing staff add additional valuable information.

The service coordinator and the Headed Home nurse review and discuss the medical records with the attending physician. *Medical considerations* that need to be part of the developmental plan are thus incorporated. These may include goals to train the family in medical caregiving responsibilities for which they lack training.

The **family** assessment may also include some written measures. These may include surveys of family needs and measures of the family's coping style. These are described more fully in Chapter 6. Further meetings with the parents serve to expand on the parents' own issues of concern and their family resources.

When the data has been gathered from the various information sources, the team reviews the information with the service coordinator. The findings are then loosely organized into major groupings. The team presents recommendations related to each member's discipline to be discussed by the service coordinator with the family.

At some point the service coordinator will work with the family in developing an **Individualized Family Service Plan (IFSP)** as required under IDEA Part H, the federal legislation mandating early intervention services. But during hospitalization, an interim plan with an agenda to complete the formal IFSP at or shortly after discharge, may be developed. This allows some intervention to begin immediately. An interim plan also gives the parents an opportunity to work on an IFSP that will be relevant when they themselves will assume primary caregiving responsibility again.

The interim plan focuses on the needs of the child and family and attempts to build on their strengths. The service coordinator provides information to the family in terms of the developmental levels determined by the Headed Home team and of the appropriate goals that might be set. The service coordinator and family work together to identify additional family goals and the relative importance the family assigns to the various goals. The family completes several surveys to assist in identifying specific needs. These are described in Chapter 6. In most instances, if a particular goal is not important to the family it is not included in the plan. The exception to this are any goals that are necessary for the medical well-being of the child.

Implementation of the Interim Intervention Plan

The developmental goals for the child and family are described in a written program. The goals are defined in functional objectives or outcomes, understandable to the family and to the medical care providers.

The plan usually addresses functional outcomes across developmental areas. Thus, goals are included for cognitive, language, motor and social functioning. Family goals, based on the parents' expressed needs, are also included. These may include assistance with problems such as obtaining transportation to the hospital or arranging a conference with a particular medical staff person.

Project Headed Home team members then participate in providing direct service to the infant and the family or in assuming a consultative role with parents and/or medical care providers. The plan is monitored through weekly team discussions. The team may make modifications in response to parent-initiated requests or developmental progress observed by the team. Changes in the child's medical status may also necessitate changes in the intervention plan.

Theoretical Basis of Project Headed Home Intervention Approaches

Educators continue to disagree on what constitutes effective intervention approaches. The target of most early intervention up to recent years has been the infant himself. Most interventions had been designed to enhance cognitive or motor development in the intervention group in contrast to a non-treated sample.

Studies of early intervention with *environmentally* at-risk populations have suggested efficacy for these approaches in terms of enhanced developmental function for the participants. The same has generally not been true of early intervention programs for *biologically* at-risk populations, such as cerebral palsy youngsters or very low birthweight prematures.

The majority of intervention approaches have been based on neurodevelopmental treatment principles. This usually involves facilitating development by preventing abnormal movement patterns from becoming habitual and by attempting to establish adaptive reflex patterns. Cognitive programs have focused on modulating stimulation to levels that are tolerable to the fragile autonomic system of at-risk infants and introducing cognitive activities appropriate to the child's developmental capabilities.

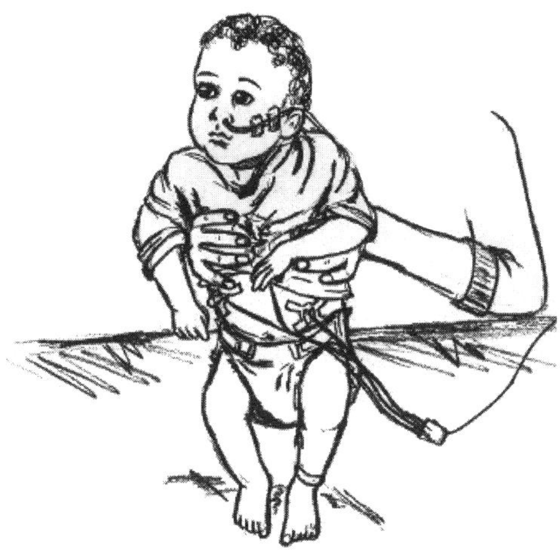

In recent years the target of intervention has expanded to include family interaction with the at-risk child. This has occurred because of the recognition that the *family is the greatest potential change agent* for the child. Parents of chronically ill children have also played an important role in voicing their perspective to policy makers, leading to philosophical changes in intervention approaches.

Maximizing infant-caregiver interaction is a major goal of several intervention theories. Familiarizing parents with the infant's cues of stress enables the caregivers to modulate their interactive behaviors so that the infant is emotionally and psychologically ready for the activity.

Another important focus of intervention has been support to the careproviders to enable them to cope with the caregiving demands of the child. While this intervention focus may not have a direct impact on enhancing the infant's IQ or motor development, it may have an important impact on the family. It may enable the family to continue to maintain their child at home. Since home-based care has been shown to be most effective for enhancing developmental potential in children with disabilities, strengthening the family's coping skills may have an important long-term effect on the child's developmental outcome.

Project Headed Home uses a synthesis of theoretical approaches, proposed by Als, et al., (1986), Barnard, et al. (1984), Gilkerson (1990), and Beckwith (1984). Facilitating opportunities for **the infant** to interact with the environment to enhance development is a major goal in the Headed Home program. Assisting **the caregiver** in understanding the various environmental factors that can enhance or hinder the infant's progress is a primary means by which it is accomplished.

For family careproviders to be in a position to address intervention techniques, they must have the following:

- Information
- Feelings of self-competence
- Minimal competing emotional demands

The Headed Home team addresses all three in serving participating families. Families learn to observe their infant's response patterns, and they receive guidance in facilitating the optimum interpersonal and environmental interaction of the infant with his world. Training, directed toward the parents, helps them see themselves as the primary interventionists on the team and feel confident about the various caregiving responsibilities they carry. Beyond this, the team, and especially the service coordinator, seek to identify, through discussions with the parents, competing needs that detract from the parents' availability to the infant. Together, they seek solutions to these other demands so the parent experiences reduced conflict.

Direct Infant Services in the PICU

Once the intervention goals have been established, the infant receives direct services from the Headed Home physical therapist and the infant specialist. Both address their respective disciplinary goals for the infant, but each one also provides a carry-over of interdisciplinary objectives. Both specialists usually plan sessions with the infant two or three times a week. In addition, the infant specialist conducts a "Baby Hour" group intervention session for all infants on the ward; the Headed Home youngsters participate when they are able.

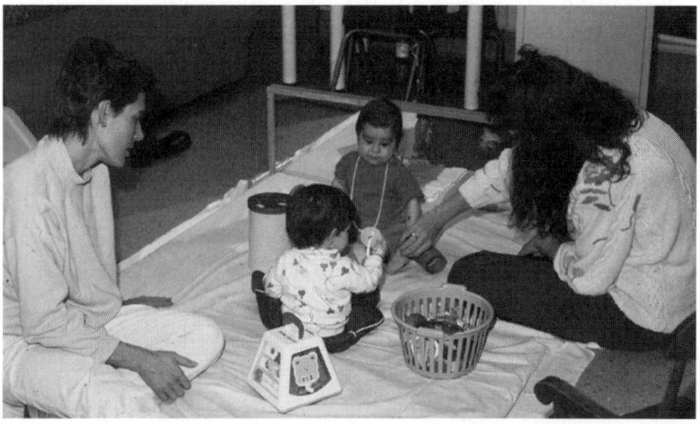

It is important that these planned sessions not compete with medical tests or procedures and vice versa. In an effort to avoid conflicts, a schedule is drawn up for each child with treatment sessions noted and discussed with the nursing staff, along with a request that procedures be scheduled at other times than the sessions. Similarly, the nurses are asked to enter the times of particular medical caregiving activities into the schedule so that intervention sessions do not conflict with them. The completed schedule is then posted at the bedside.

As often as possible, sessions are planned for times when the parents can participate. Giving the parents direct guidance in intervention techniques is the best method for developing confidence in their own abilities to provide developmental activities. However, some parents whose children have long stays in the hospital are able to visit only in the evening or early morning. The Headed Home team members make special arrangements to meet with the family at some of those times. When the parents are not able to meet frequently, other communication strategies are employed, including the following:

- Regular telephone contact
- Home visits
- A list of weekly goals and activities posted at the bedside
- A communication book

Communication with Parents

A regular dialogue with parents is essential. The needs of the family may change from week to week. Parents may need clarification of goals and activities. The strategies mentioned above are all utilized in maintaining this dialogue. The **activity sheets** posted by the bed are regularly updated. They include a photograph of the child during a particular activity. An example of the format used for the activity sheet is shown in Chapter 4, Figure F "This week I'm working on...."

The **communication book** is perhaps the most important means by which the staff and parents maintain an information exchange. The book usually includes daily comments inserted by the parents and the Headed Home staff. It usually includes photographs of the child, showing her progress. The book serves as an ongoing chronicle of the child's development over time and becomes a valuable record to the parents.

Home visitation by hospital staff has special meaning to parents. It allows them to interact with the professional staff on their "territory." It allows for more personal contact than can be achieved in the institutional facility. Home visits take on a particular importance as discharge planning begins. Knowledge of the physical and psychosocial aspects of the home situation is essential in developing ways to integrate the child into the family unit at home.

Communication with Medical /Nursing Caregivers

After the family, communication with **medical/nursing caregivers** is the next most important aspect for the effective carry-over of the intervention plan. Regular communication with the nurses who care for the child provides an avenue for two-way communication. The nurses who are with the child the most time are in a position to integrate developmental goals into the medical caregiving plan. Nurses' observations may be highly informative in determining the infant's response style and interactive capability during the acute illness.

Regular face-to-face discussion with some of the nurses responsible for the child is essential, but it may be difficult because of their rotation schedule. When this is the case, Headed Home team members use similar strategies to those described for the family to maintain dialogue with the nurses. If oral-motor functioning effects feeding, the Headed Home speech pathologist consults with the nurse to observe the feeding strategies being utilized. The speech pathologist makes specific recommendations to the nurses as to the techniques to employ, leaving pictures and if necessary, a video demonstration. The service coordinator or another team member may then explore these techniques with the family and introduce them into the management plan.

Periodically, meetings that include the parents, the relevant hospital physician, a primary nurse, the ward social worker, the service coordinator and sometimes other members of the Headed Home team are held to furnish an updating on the child's progress from various standpoints. Such meetings provide a valuable time for information to be integrated for the family. They also allow an opportunity for delegating necessary tasks to the appropriate staff member so all the child and family needs are met.

The Intervention Activities for the Infant

Activities planned for the child generally address the developmental areas of:

- Cognitive development
- Speech-language development/oral motor functioning

- Gross and fine motor skills
- Psychosocial functioning

Activities are selected that will be enjoyable for the infant and the caregiver. Whenever possible, they are designed to be incorporated into a regular caregiving activity. For example, work on fine motor skills might be incorporated into feeding time by encouraging finger feeding. Activities must often be adapted to the medical status of the child on a particular day.

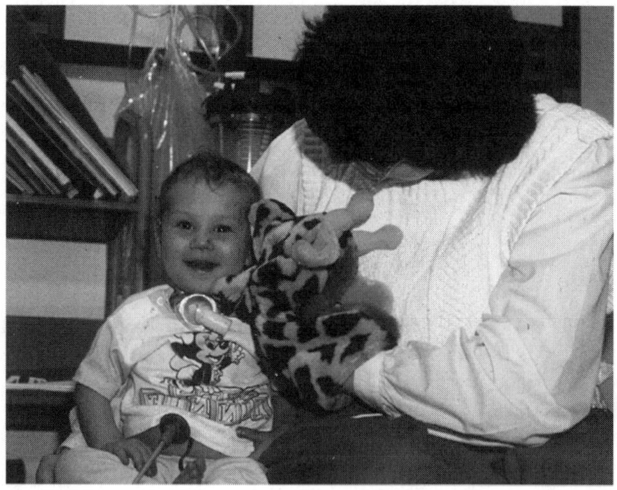

Some chronically ill children are very distressed when they are handled by individuals other than their family. This is sometimes the consequence of many invasive procedures the child has been exposed to during necessary medical interventions. When this is the case, the team members should train and encourage the family members to carry out as much of the intervention plan as possible. At the same time, team members and other non-family members can attempt to desensitize the child to social overtures. Talking, singing, and introducing toys while, at the same time, staff avoid touching the child, may serve to reduce his anxiety and allow positive interaction experiences to occur.

Specific goals and activities utilized in the program are described in Chapter 4.

Discharge Planning

As the child's medical condition begins to stabilize, preparation of the family, the home, and necessary community services intensifies in readiness for discharge. In fact, a truly effective discharge plan begins early in the hospital stay.

For parents of children participating in the Headed Home program, the specific areas in which they need training will have been identified and addressed on an ongoing basis. This is a positive consequence of maintaining a focus on the parent as the primary care provider. As the discharge period nears, the Headed Home team reviews additional training needs and identifies the community services needed. Usually a discharge planning meeting is held with the following people among those participating:

- Attending physician
- Headed Home service coordinator
- Specialty physicians and nurse specialist
- Social worker
- Family
- Discharge nurse

The social worker and the discharge nurse generally assume responsibility for coordinating the medical services needed after discharge. The Headed Home team coordinates developmental services, and the team nurse provides home visits to the family prior to and following the discharge to identify additional home care needs and to facilitate the ease of management in the home setting.

A list of arrangements that must be completed and services that must be in place before discharge is usually developed. Each need is assigned to a particular member of the team who is then responsible for its completion by a designated date.

A day or so before discharge another meeting is arranged to be sure that all services are in place at home and in the community. Medications and the medical follow-up plan are reviewed.

On the day of discharge, the service coordinator and the Headed Home nurse remain in phone contact with the family; one of them plans several home visits during the immediate post-discharge period.

Management of Home Care

The Headed Home team reevaluates the family's training and service needs after home care begins because the reality of care may be different from what was anticipated during discharge planning. Some children make dramatic improvements in such areas as feeding or in respiratory status once they are home. Usually two to three weeks after discharge, the service coordinator visits the family at home for a discussion to formalize an Individualized Family Service Plan (IFSP) if one has not been completed earlier. If a prior IFSP exists, the service coordinator takes this opportunity to update that plan. The service coordinator conducts this interview with a relatively open format but guides the discussion so that the family is able to identify its strengths and concerns. Once the needs have been identified, the family determines the order of importance in which those concerns will be addressed.

A multitude of medical/nursing services may be required to maintain the child in the home setting. When a problem with the provision of these services arises, the service coordinator and the Headed Home nurse assist the family in solving the difficulties. They may help the family solve problems with home nursing care agencies or resolve conflicting recommendations from different medical specialists.

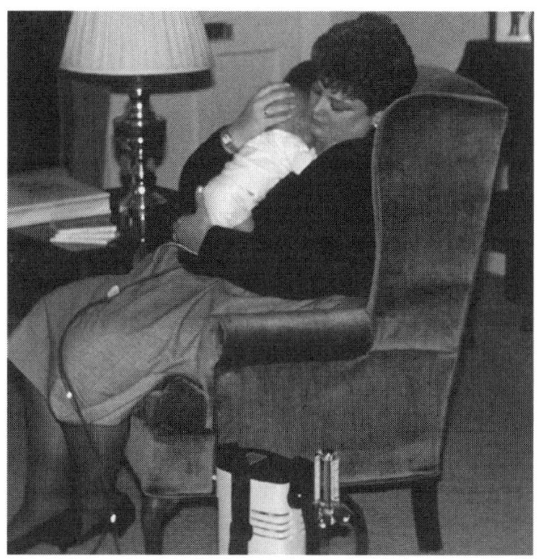

The Headed Home service coordinator also serves as a liaison with community-based early intervention services for which the child and her family may be eligible. The service coordinator and family bring the child to the attention of the local agency responsible for the delivery of infant intervention under IDEA Part H. The assessment information gathered by the Headed Home team is often used by the agency to determine eligibility for services.

The majority of children participating in Project Headed Home remain medically fragile in the period following discharge and must be provided a **home-based** early intervention program. Many communities are now developing home-based early intervention teams trained to work with children with chronic medical conditions. The Headed Home team works with these personnel in developing an appropriate intervention plan for the child and family. Headed Home team members provide direct training to community personnel, when special training is needed to manage an aspect of the child's daily care needs. Their goal is to provide a smooth transition from the Headed Home intervention plan to the community-based intervention team's plan.

A very critical area of need for most families in the post-discharge period is for emotional support. At times individual counseling may be beneficial for parents and/or siblings to help them deal with the stresses of managing the child at home. If the parents themselves are the primary caregivers and are without home nursing relief, then perhaps respite care to relieve them of their continuous caregiving burden will be the most vital need.

The Headed Home team maintains frequent contact with the family during this period, so that the family's needs are addressed as they arise. Once services are in place and the child's condition remains stable, responsibility for coordination of services begins to shift to the community-based agencies.

Rehospitalization

It is anticipated that at times the chronically ill child will need rehospitalization either for surgical revisions or during acute illness. As time goes by, the hope is that these hospitalizations will diminish in frequency and in length. When rehospitalization is required, the Headed Home team again assesses the child's need for intervention and the family needs as a whole that must be addressed during the rehospitalization. The Headed Home service coordinator secures information from community-based service providers for the child. This information allows the Headed Home team to continue the goals of the community-based intervention plan during hospitalization without prolonged interruption if the child's medical condition permits. The Headed Home team's familiarity with the child's developmental needs also assures that continuity in developmental programming can be maintained during the hospital stay. Once again the service coordinator works with the family at the time of discharge to be sure all the needed services are in place. The service coordinator remains available to the family to assist with these issues until the medical problems resolve or a member of the community-based intervention team is able to assume that role.

Providing Family Support

The service coordinators of infants enrolled in Project Headed Home often develop a particularly close relationship with the family of the chronically ill child. The service coordinator, unlike most of the hospital staff, is in a position to visit with the family at home, to talk with them regularly on the phone, and to have contact with community service providers for the family.

The service coordinator frequently becomes an important emotional support for the family. Families use the service coordinator as a sounding board for the frustrations they experience in dealing with complex health and social systems. They may even discuss family conflicts over decision-making about particular issues.

It may be that a service coordinator represents a discipline that has not emphasized skills in family counseling as part of the professional training. The reality of early intervention, however, is that a family may grow to depend on a particular intervention team member even though that person may not be a social service provider. The Headed Home model acknowledges that this is a situation likely to develop and attempts to strengthen the social support skills of members of the team as needed. The Headed Home psychologist provides guidance to the service coordinator in supportive strategies for the family. This does not mean the service coordinator provides a formal counseling relationship; instead, the service coordinator is a person who is a supportive listener and an information resource. For families who need professional counseling, the service coordinator assists them in identifying an appropriate resource.

In a number of instances, a particular family has tried to establish a more personal social relationship with the service coordinator or another team member. When this has meant invitations to join family celebrations related to the child, the staff member usually accepts. By inviting the interventionist to lunch at the home, the child's mother may want to reciprocate for what she recognizes as genuine caring by the service coordinator. Team members are generally comfortable in responding to something like that. But at other times, the service coordinator may recognize that the parent is seeking a closer social relationship as a replacement for broader peer contact. In these instances, the service coordinator tries to help the parent expand her individual and group social involvement. Chapter 7 provides a fuller discussion of the service coordinator's role in providing family support.

Perhaps the most difficult aspect of the Headed Home model is the necessity of supporting families through the death of the child. This is an unfortunate reality of work with a medically fragile population. About one-third of the children originally identified to participate in the program died before their second birthdays. Even though the fact that the child remains at high risk of death despite periods of relative stability is in the back of everyone's mind, it is none the less devastating to both family and team members when the child dies. Perhaps the level of hope that a family must maintain in order to get through each day is what requires some repression of the reality of the child's fragility. It is also the children themselves, who can be so alive and engaging while they go through a stable period, that make one believe that their status will only improve.

In a number of instances, members of the Headed Home team were asked by the family to be with them as their child was dying. One family was comforted by the fact that their service coordinator arrived in the room just before the child died so the child had a chance to see her "special friend" once more. At memorial services, project staff often spoke, highlighting some very unique characteristic of the child and her family.

As with counseling, many team members have not been prepared in their disciplinary role to help families with bereavement. And yet the family may count on the service coordinator or other therapist for support at this time. The Headed Home team works closely with the hospital nursing staff in following particular procedures at the time of the death of an infant to provide support to the family. Details of the procedures followed are included in Chapter 7.

What was learned through the Headed Home model is that disciplinary role division may not be very important when it comes to family support. The family usually finds one particular team member with whom they relate more easily than others. That person is then naturally the one the family turns to for support. As a result, that individual may need guidance as to how best to meet the needs of the family.

One of the most effective aspects of the Headed Home model is its goal to support families in their variety of needs. In many cases, early intervention is not going to "cure" the child. The child may have such significant disability that developmental gains may be small despite early intervention. What the project does achieve is that it helps families to cope and even to grow despite almost unimaginably difficult circumstances.

Transition into Community Services

The Headed Home model was intended to serve children from birth to three years of age. The project was designed particularly to assist the families of medically fragile infants whose children had not yet been brought to the attention of community-based intervention providers. Secondly, the project targeted children who were already involved in community-based programs but who needed continuity in intervention during hospitalizations. An integral part of the program, however, is the collaborative interchange between the hospital-based services and those within the community. The intention of the Headed Home team is that their involvement diminishes as the child's medical condition stabilizes and as community supports are well in place.

In the majority of instances, children reach this point between ages two and three. By this time, children with respiratory compromise are usually more stable, at least in warmer months. For those children with congenital defects, corrective surgeries have often been accomplished by this time and their medical status has improved. Revisions of the IFSP developed with the Headed Home program would have continued to reflect this shift in capability. As services have expanded in the community in response to IDEA Part H, other supports and even other service coordinators are available to assist families negotiate systems to have their needs served. The Headed Home team is prepared to communicate their knowledge about the child and family to these service providers as it assists in the smooth transition of the child and family into this new domain. This may mean visiting a prospective school with the family to help the staff in that facility feel comfortable in meeting the needs of the child. It often means encouraging discussion between agencies in the community for greater collaboration in serving the family's needs. The Headed Home team achieves success in meeting its goals when its role is completely assumed by appropriate community services.

Adaptation of the Model

This discussion has focused on how a particular early intervention model can be conducted in a hospital PICU. This program was designed in keeping with the administrative structure and staffing patterns characteristic of Georgetown University Hospital, a tertiary care center. Administrative and staffing patterns will certainly differ in some ways in other settings. Nevertheless, this model, or elements of it, can be adapted to fit other hospital structures. Health care professionals from disciplines other than those represented on the Headed Home team might also be appropriate for some aspects of service provision. Social workers, pediatric nurse practitioners, and occupational therapists could fulfill some of the responsibilities assumed by other professionals in the Headed Home model. It may be helpful to have one member of the team who has particular credibility with the medical staff of the PICU and another who has the confidence of the nursing staff play an active role in the introduction of an intervention program to these staff members. Some physicians may be skeptical about the intent and effectiveness of early intervention, as well as protective of the families they serve. The steps needed to establish or maintain the confidence of the physician in the program include these:

- Personal meetings
- Providing background literature on similar programs
- Maintaining close contact to secure approval for programming for each identified child

- Providing regular feedback on the progress of particular children

In a hospital, it is usually the nursing staff who are instrumental in seeing that program goals are actually carried out. Therefore, obtaining the interest and support of nurses is essential to the program's success. Nurses have become increasingly interested in understanding the negative consequences of hospitalization on developing young children. They may be eager for further information about what roles they may play in an early intervention provision on the inpatient services. A number of video materials have recently been developed (Pokorni, 1990, 1992) that may be helpful in preparing the staff to incorporate developmental goals into caregiving plans. The video format is helpful because it is usually very difficult to get nurses together as a group, due to their staff responsibility. Videotapes allow greater self-study flexibility.

CONCLUSION

With expansion of both service needs and federal mandates for early intervention for chronically ill infants, more hospitals will be seeking ways to incorporate a developmental component to care plans for these at-risk children. Project Headed Home offers a comprehensive model particularly targeted at meeting the needs of the infant's family as a whole. The complexities of this population of young children will require close collaboration of medical and developmental staff both within and outside the hospital. Hospital-based personnel will have an increasing need to be aware of the variety of community-based services necessary to monitor the child at home. It is only through this collaborative effort that families of chronically ill infants will be able to deal with the many stresses of caring for their children. Hopefully, successful collaboration will also contribute to improved outcome for these vulnerable children.

REFERENCES

Als, H., Lawhon, G., Brown, E., Gibes, R., Duffy, F., McAnulty, G., & Blickman, J. (1986). Individualized behavioral and environmental care for the very low birth weight preterm infant at high risk for bronchopulmonary dysplasia: Neonatal intensive care unit and developmental outcome *Pediatrics, 78,* 1123-1132.

Barnard, K., Bee, H., & Hammond, M. (1984). Developmental changes in maternal interactions with term and preterm infants. *Infant Behavior and Development, 7,* 101-113.

Beckwith, L. (1984). Parent interaction with their preterm infants and later mental development. *Early Childhood Development and Care, 16,* 27-40.

Gilkerson, L. (1990). Understanding institutional functioning style: A resource for hospital/early intervention collaboration. *Infants and Young Children,* 2(3), 22-30.

Pokorni, J. (1990). *Developmental intervention for hospitalized infants.* Boston, MA: Polymorph Films.

Pokorni, J. (1992). *Infants in transitional care: A videotape series for professionals working with young children in chronic care facilities.* Lawrence, KS: Learner Managed Designs, Inc.

Chapter 4

Early Intervention for Hospitalized Infants on the Pediatric Intensive Care Unit

Cynthia Baker, M.A. and Kathleen A. Shapiro, P.T.

Pediatric Intensive Care has evolved dramatically over the past decade, as the active intervention and successful treatment of young infants has produced increased survival. Intensive care for infants has focused heavily on the support of the newborn low birth weight infant served within a Neonatal Intensive Care Unit (NICU). NICUs are designed primarily to provide special care to the **premature** newborn infant in the acute phase of illness following delivery. They remain hospitalized for a significant period of time until the point at which they are stable enough to be discharged to their homes.

With recent advances in medical support and technology, many infants who in the past would not have lived are now surviving, albeit with chronic medical problems that require continued hospitalization, sometimes for weeks or even months. Despite medical instability, these infants, as they mature, begin to demonstrate increased periods of alertness and the capability to interact with their surroundings. The NICU is not an appropriate environment for the long-term care of these infants even though they continue to require intensive medical support. The infants may physically outgrow the equipment designed for neonates. Many require rehospitalization after they are discharged home, but hospitals generally do not accept admissions to the newborn unit for these patients.

The older premature infant who continues to require intensive medical support is usually transferred to a **pediatric intensive care unit (PICU)**. The PICU is also the site of care for another 4 percent of infants who are born at full term with complications that require specialized care in the early months of life (Ballard, 1988). These complications may include neonatal asphyxia, congenital anomalies, neurological abnormalities, or infection. Among the necessary medical interventions for these infants are ventilation, tracheotomy, shunt placement, surgical repair, and intravenous therapy. Daily caregiving needs include frequent suctioning, respiratory therapy, frequent blood drawing to obtain blood gases, tube feeding (nasogastric or g-tube), transfusion, infusion, surgical site care, and basic infant care and bathing. A new specialization then, of *Pediatric Intensive Care,* has become necessary to appropriately meet the needs of these chronically ill infants and their families (Richardson & Robinson, 1989).

This section will focus on early intervention provided within the PICU. While considerable attention has been focused on the NICU (Als et al., 1986), little has been described about needs of infants in the PICU.

DIFFERENCES BETWEEN THE NICU AND PICU ENVIRONMENTS

The NICU

Medical intervention for an infant in the NICU differs in many ways from that in the PICU. The primary focus of the NICU staff and environment is on the infant's survival. Little thought may be given to long-term outcome expectations at this time. The major focus is to get the infant through each day. A secondary goal is for the NICU infant to attain medical stability. This may take from several weeks to several months. The infant is constantly at risk for infections, which almost always produce a setback. Many infants have trouble weaning off the ventilator and need to be reintubated and extubated several times before they learn to breathe fully on their own. A third goal of the NICU team is to have the infant grow and mature both physiologically and developmentally. Again, this may take a considerable amount of time as the infant is challenged to learn to:

- Maintain an appropriate body temperature
- Control his breathing patterns
- Feed adequately from a nipple in order to gain weight consistently

Developmental intervention may be introduced at this time, focusing primarily on:

- Positioning of the infant to reduce abnormal postures
- Finding ways to reduce the infant's stress in response to procedures
- Providing some simple developmental activities, usually in the form of appropriate social and sensory stimulation

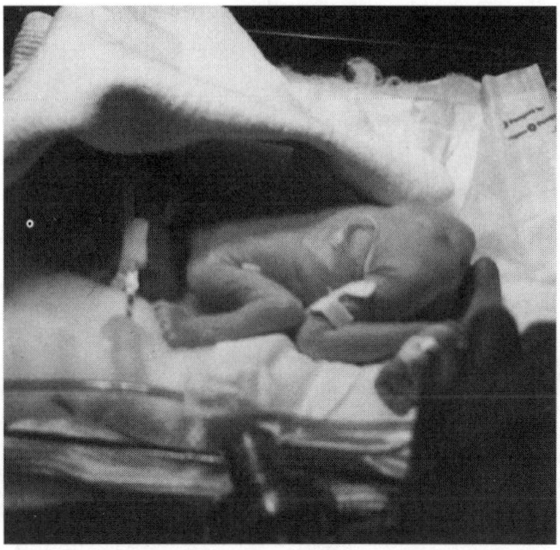

Due to the acute nature of the infant's medical condition, these interventions must often be postponed or, at best, incorporated to some extent by the primary nurse while attending to the infant's medical needs.

While the infant in the NICU may have limited periods of alertness, she remains predominantly "tuned out" or in a light sleep, unavailable for interaction. These infants are lethargic, listless, and have difficulty attending to and assimilating sensory input from their environment. This makes it difficult for these infants and their caregivers to establish meaningful interaction.

Families of infants in the NICU often feel overwhelmed by the level of medical technology and unfamiliar terminology to which they are suddenly exposed. Parents may go through a period when they have difficulty forming an attachment to their infant; they may distance themselves for self-protection in the fear that their child will die (Ballard, 1988). This is exacerbated by the fact that parents may be provided only a limited caregiving role for their very ill infant due to the complex medical caregiving needs.

The PICU

Usually the PICU is physically a larger medical unit than the NICU and serves a broader age range of children from infancy to adolescence who evidence a variety of medical conditions. Some children in the PICU require hospitalization secondary to:

- Childhood illnesses, such as leukemia, cystic fibrosis, and asthma
- Emergencies, such as drowning, car accidents, child abuse or other unanticipated trauma

The majority of other patients in the birth to three years of age range will be NICU "graduates" who are:

- Transferred to the PICU for extended medical care
- Rehospitalized following discharge from the NICU
- Full-term infants with perinatal complications

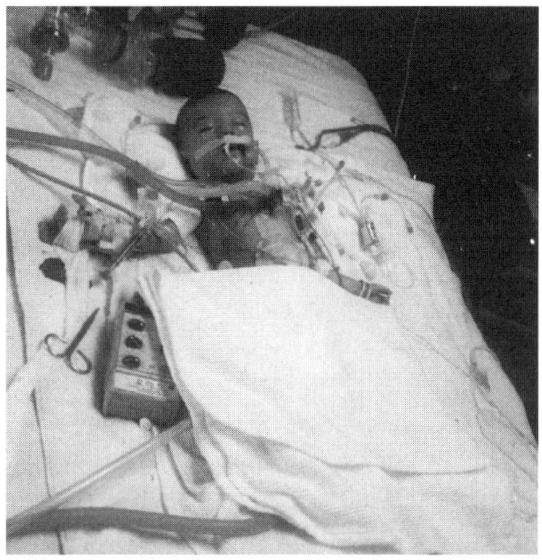

The infant in the PICU tends to be more mature and stable physiologically than the neonate. The crisis-oriented focus of "lifesaving" is not as continuous as in the NICU, although in any PICU there are children who are very ill. More often, the PICU infant is in an acute or chronic state of illness which requires continual monitoring and caregiving. The greater level of maturity in PICU infants is often associated with greater body weight; therefore, they demonstrate increased physical stamina and decreased fragility. Their respiratory capacity tends to be more stable than the NICU infants', and the onset of acute problems, such as apnea and bradycardia, is more predictable. The exception is the NICU graduate who is transferred to the PICU for long-term respiratory support and care. She is often ventilator-dependent for some time and may require tracheotomy.

The PICU infant tends to have longer periods of alertness that are also of better quality than the NICU infant. This is most obvious in the infant whose condition is chronic yet stable. These infants' caregiving needs stay somewhat consistent from day to day, and they require fewer regular intrusive medical procedures. These children have increased capacity to respond to and learn from their environment. Often, providing intervention to these infants enhances their state of alertness, further increasing their availability to learn.

The role of the family of infants on the PICU also expands from what it was in the NICU. Typically, they have had more opportunities to develop an attachment to the infant, and their initial fear of the infant's imminent death has been reduced. The PICU environment generally offers parents a chance to assume a more primary caregiving role for the infant. For the infant who has already been at home with the family, her parents may wish to play a more active role in making decisions concerning her medical care. In turn, the child is more responsive to the family. Understandably, infants who have been in the home environment may be at risk for emotional distress upon being separated from the family. Strategies for optimizing the infant's psychosocial well-being and continued bonding with the family despite continuing needs for hospitalization are needed.

ORGANIZATION OF THE PICU

A typical PICU is an active unit centered around one or more nursing stations and treatment rooms. Units vary in size from a few to as many as 50 beds. There are usually both single and double patient rooms, and at least one or two rooms are designated as strictly isolation rooms for patients with highly infectious illnesses. In recent years, "mini units" with six to eight beds in one larger room (often termed Special Care Units) have been used for young patients requiring chronic care or a rehabilitative focus of care (Cole, 1989). These units may be fashioned into "homelike" environments, affording more opportunity for interaction among children and a less institutional atmosphere. A room may be available for a family to gather together, as well as a staffed and accessible playroom. Siblings may be permitted, if they are healthy, to visit with the hospitalized child.

The units are staffed by physicians, nurses, unit secretaries, technicians, and respiratory therapists. In teaching hospitals and universities, there are the additional fellows, residents, medical students and student nurses. Also working on a unit at any time will be social workers, nutritionists, pastoral care staff, physical, occupational, and speech therapists, developmental specialists, pediatric psychologists, child-life specialists, and housekeeping staff. Ancillary professionals, such as medical subspecialists or X-ray personnel, typically see patients on a consultant basis as the need arises. Figure D provides a schematic perspective of PICU staffing. Rarely is a unit quiet, especially during weekdays. Confusion is common for families and children exposed to this myriad of professionals with differing roles.

Figure D
Organization of PICU Staff

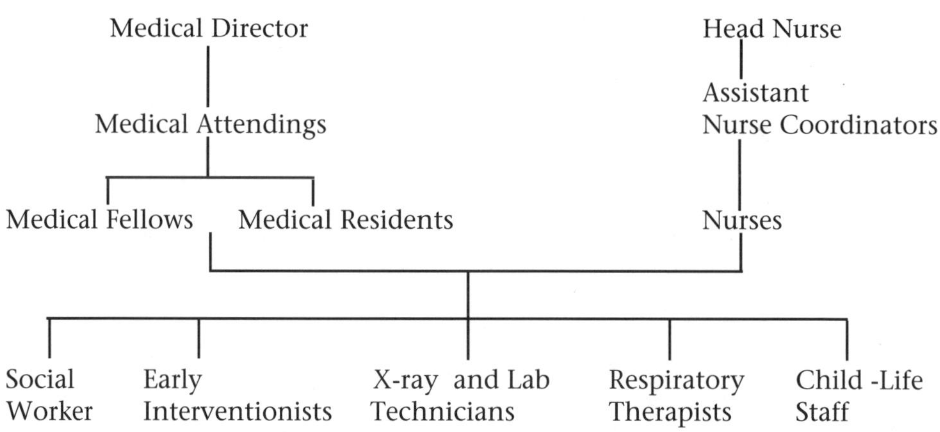

Pediatric units vary as to their staffing and shift patterns. A **primary nursing system** is optimal for patients and families. With this pattern, each child is assigned to a specific nurse for the duration of the child's hospital course. During this nurse's shifts on the unit, he or she is responsible for the nursing care of that child. This approach is advantageous in the following ways:

- The infant or child becomes familiar with one primary medical caregiver.
- The family relies on a consistent and informed source of communication concerning their child.
- The nurse becomes familiar with the child and her particular needs.

Unfortunately, this method of staffing has become less feasible since nursing schedules have shifted from five eight-hour workdays, to three twelve-hour workdays. The result is that several different nurses are assigned to a child during the week.

Continuity of care for patients is difficult in light of scheduling patterns, per diem nurses, and day-to-day changes in patient census on the ward. To enhance communication among the unit staff, weekly "Family Rounds" or "Child-Life Rounds" are often a regular PICU activity, so that various disciplines involved with each child and family can share information and agree on optimal approaches towards intervention and care for each child. Nursing coordinators must continually devise communication strategies for the nursing staff so the individual needs of children and families on the unit are recognized and integrated by all of the staff into daily caregiving.

ASSESSING DEVELOPMENTAL NEEDS OF PICU PATIENTS

Children identified as potentially in need of therapeutic or early intervention services on an inpatient unit must be evaluated to establish their baseline skills. It may be difficult to obtain accurate developmental information for assessing hospitalized infants and toddlers because the child may be too sick to respond optimally. The hospital environment itself is hardly conducive to a child's best performance even when his medical condition is stable. This must be taken into account when using assessments for purposes of predicting later ability.

The assessment process may require two phases:

1) An initial determination of a child's current levels of functioning in various developmental skill areas
2) An ongoing process to identify:
   - The child's unique needs and availability for intervention
   - The nature and extent of services to be provided
   - The family's strengths and needs during and after hospitalization

   (Fewell, 1991)

INFORMAL ASSESSMENT

The overall philosophy concerning assessment of a hospitalized infant is that it is an evolving process. Often changes occur in a baby's status and mood from morning to afternoon, and certainly from day to day. Professionals working with hospitalized infants should conduct a quick, informal, daily assessment of each infant prior to any intervention. The following provides a guideline for daily assessment:

- What is the baby's current medical status?
- What are the behavioral effects of current medications on the infant (drowsiness, irritability, nausea)?
- Has the infant has adequate sleep in the past 24 hours?
- Has the infant had adequate food intake in the past 24 hours?
- What are the physical limitations of the infant due to medical interventions (placement and number of I.V.s, feeding pumps, respiratory supports, positional requirements for shunt drainage or reflux)?
- What is the infant's capacity for alertness?
- How much involvement has the infant had with family members in the past 24 hours?

- How does the baby respond to social and play interaction?

Information derived from an informal assessment may prove very helpful in determining a child's status and present availability for intervention activities.

FORMAL ASSESSMENT

Formal assessment of a baby should be conducted only when she is at an optimal state mentally and physically. If at all possible, it is best to schedule the evaluation when the parents can be present. Which measures to select depends on the age of the infant, her medical status, and her existing skills. Certainly, no single test or tool should be the only source of information used in the multidisciplinary evaluation of a child. The following tools are available for use with the infant/toddler and preschool population. They should only be administered by trained professionals.

NEONATAL ASSESSMENT MEASURES

Brazelton Neonatal Behavioral Assessment Scale (NBAS) (Brazelton, 1984) is a behavioral exam for the infant between 37 and 44 weeks gestation. Seven response patterns are assessed: habituation, orientation, motor, range of states, regulation of state, autonomic regulation and reflexes.

Assessment of Premature Infant Behavior (APIB) was developed by Als et al. (1982) to assess signs of infant stress and self-regulation. Scoring is time-consuming, and extensive training with the test's developers is perceived to be necessary for valid administration.

Naturalistic Observation of Newborn Behavior (Als, 1984) is a procedure based on the APIB, but the infant's responses to stress and support from the environment do not require handling of the infant as does the APIB. The infant is observed for behavior responses during caregiving procedures.

The Neurological Assessment of the Preterm and Full-Term Infant (Dubowitz and Dubowitz, 1981) provides observations of the posture, tone of the trunk and extremities, primitive reflexes, and habituation of the infant. It is designed to be administered from three days to term age.

COGNITIVE AND GENERAL DEVELOPMENTAL MEASURES

Infant /Toddler Scales

Bayley Scales of Infant Development (Bayley, 1969) is the most widely used, nationally standardized test of cognitive and motor ability for infants and toddlers. This tool is comprised of both a mental development and psychomotor scale. An infant behavior record is provided to record social, temperamental and behavioral aspects of an infant's performance. The mental scale includes items and tasks relating to social responsiveness, fine motor ability, object permanence, problem solving, visual-perceptual tasks, and language. The psychomotor scale tests skills of both fine motor development and gross motor development. The test is well normed and numerical scores (mental developmental index and psychomotor index) are derived along with age equivalents of the infant's skills. A revision with updated norms will be released in the near future. The test may be used with children functioning in the one-month to thirty-month range.

Revised Gesell Developmental Schedules (Knobloch, et al., 1980) served as the foundation for most of the other scales in use today. The test provides assessment of four domains, including motor, language, personal-social, and adaptive. It may be used for children functioning at levels from one month to six years.

Griffiths' Mental Development Scales (Griffiths, 1976) is designed for use from birth to eight years. It is comprised of scales measuring skill areas including locomotor, personal-social, hearing and speech, eye and hand coordination, and performance. A general developmental quotient may be obtained as well as age equivalents for each of the sub-scales. Although normed on a British sample, the items appear appropriate for American children although scores on the Griffiths appear higher than those achieved on the Bayley (Ramsay and Fitzhardinge, 1977).

Infant Psychological Development Scales (Uzgiris and Hunt, 1975) is a criterion-referenced test of whose findings may be translated into intervention goals more easily than with the norm-referenced tests mentioned above. It is based on Piaget developmental stage theory.

Callier-Azusa Scale (Stillman, 1978) is a developmental rating scale that allows assessment of children with multiple or severe disabilities including deaf-blind. It evaluates performance across sub-scales of motor development; perceptual development; daily living skills; cognition, communication and language, and social development. It can be used for individuals functioning from birth to nine years.

Reynell-Zinkin Scales (Reynell, 1979) is an assessment tool for visually impaired young children functioning in the birth to five-year range with separate norm tables for sighted, partially sighted, and blind children. The items tap object manipulation, object permanence, and environmental exploration, independent of vision.

Other tools that are useful in the evaluation of infants and toddlers are those that are more curriculum-focused and usually allow for multi-domain evaluation. These are advantageous for many reasons. They are relatively inexpensive in comparison with some of the more normatively-based tools; they can be administered by staff with more limited testing experience; and they frequently come with curriculum packages that can be part of the intervention plan. The tests often span a fairly wide age range, and the same test may be administered repeatedly to the same infant.

Hawaii Early Learning Profile (HELP) (Furuno et al., 1984) is a curriculum-based evaluation that uses a comprehensive multi-item checklist in each of six domains: cognitive, expressive language, fine motor, gross motor, social-emotional, and self-help. This evaluation gives a broad age range level of functioning in each separate domain so that strengths and weaknesses across domains can be derived. It is accompanied by both curriculum and parent-focused practical materials for planning and intervention that addresses each skill item.

Carolina Curriculum for Handicapped Infants and Infants at Risk (Johnson-Martin, N., Jens, K., & Attermeier, S., 1986), a curriculum-based evaluation, is built on normal sequences of development and logical teaching sequences and is designed specifically for use with infants with disabilities. An assessment log, consisting of 24 curriculum sequences, allows for evaluation of skills in a wide range of areas. Teaching activities and intervention strategies are provided for each of the items.

Preschool Scales

For children functioning above the two-and a half-year level, it is possible to administer one of the well-standardized formal IQ measures. These tests offer greater predictive validity than measures used in infancy.

McCarthy Scales of Children's Abilities (McCarthy, 1972) is designed for children between the ages of two and a half to eight and a half years. It yields a profile of abilities, including verbal, perceptual-performance, quantitative, memory and motor scale scores. A general cognitive index (GCI) is also calculated.

Stanford Binet Intelligence Scale (4th edition) (Thorndike et al. 1986) provides assessment in sub-scales of verbal reasoning, abstract visual reasoning, quantitative reasoning and short-term memory. Standard age scores are calculated for each sub-scale as well as a composite score. This revision is less weighted towards verbal abilities than the previous edition. It is designed for use with children ages two years up to twenty-three years.

Kaufman Assessment Battery for Children (K-ABC) (Kaufman & Kaufman, 1983) is designed for children ages two and a half to twelve and a half. It consists of two major scales—the sequential processing scale and the simultaneous processing scale—and also yields a mental-processing composite (MPC). It was developed with the intent of having a measure more culturally fair to children from disadvantaged backgrounds. The test is very visually based and includes a procedure for scoring based on nonverbal sub-tests only.

Merrill-Palmer Scale of Mental Tests (Stutsman, 1931) is a primarily nonverbal measure for children functioning in the cognitive range of eighteen months to six years. While lacking current normative standardization, the test is useful with nonverbal preschoolers, particularly those with pervasive developmental disorder.

NEUROMOTOR MEASURES

The Infant Motor Screen (Nickel et al., 1989) was designed to provide early neuromotor diagnosis of infants at risk for cerebral palsy. It is designed for infants from four to sixteen months corrected age. It assesses muscle tone, primitive reflexes, automatic reactions, and asymmetries. This scale is adapted from two earlier infant neuromotor tests: the Milani-Comparetti (Pearson, 1975) and the Movement Assessment of Infants (Chandler et al, 1980).

Peabody Developmental Motor Scales (Folio and Fewell, 1983) is a gross and fine motor evaluation measure for children from birth to eighty-three months.

SPEECH AND LANGUAGE MEASURES

Speech and language measures for infants usually include administration procedures that provide for scoring by observed performance and by parent report. (See Chapter 5 for additional suggestions for language assessment.)

Receptive-Expressive Emergent Language Scale (REEL) (Bzoch and League, 1991) provides a receptive language age, an expressive language age, and a combined language age. It can be used with children from birth to three years.

Sequenced Inventory of Communication Development - Revised (SICD-R) (Hedrick et al., 1984). Extensive reliance on parent report and limited items below twenty-four months make this somewhat less useful for developmentally delayed infants and toddlers, although it is described as appropriate for children from four months to four years.

Reynell Developmental Language Scale (Reynell, 1977) measures verbal comprehension and expressive language skills both by parent report and observation. It is designed for use with children from one to seven years.

SOCIAL-EMOTIONAL BEHAVIOR MEASURES

Vineland Adaptive Behavior Scale (Sparrow et al., 1984) provides an assessment of social interaction and adaptive skills from infancy to adulthood. Scoring is by report of the caregiver. Additional sub-scales include communication and motor scales.

Bayley Infant Behavior Record (Bayley, 1969) is a clinical observation tool scored during Bayley Mental and Motor Scale administration. Provides information on the child's attentional style and interactive capabilities.

Carolina Record of Infant Behavior (CRIB) (Simeonsson et al., 1982) is an observational measure of children at the sensorimotor level of development. It provides an evaluation of the infant's state and capability for interaction with individuals and the environment.

With very medically fragile infants, an assessment may best be accomplished using a transdisciplinary format, so as not to overtax the infant. The physical therapist should assist in positioning the infant appropriately while another team member administers test items directly to the infant. The remaining team members may then help suggest tasks for evaluation of performance and record the infant's responses. Assignment of these roles depends on the age of the child and his primary developmental needs. It is important to continually monitor the infant's medical status and stress signals, and to remain sensitive to the infant's capacity for interaction during the assessment. It may be necessary to complete the evaluation over the course of two or three sessions.

ASSESSING FAMILY NEEDS

In the past, the focus of early intervention has been on the infant alone or the parent-infant interaction. The currently regarded "best practice" is to view the infant's needs *within the context of the family* as a whole. Towards this end, assessment is made of the strengths and particular concerns expressed by an individual family. A part of the initial evaluation process, the assessment is accomplished through a variety of strategies (McGonigel et al., 1991).

In the situation of a family whose child is hospitalized for what is anticipated as a limited amount of time, this process may be accomplished best in two stages. In the first stage, an intervention team member, service coordinator, or hospital social worker meets with the family shortly after the child's hospitalization The purpose of the meeting is to discuss their perspectives on the needs of their child and problems in other aspects of family life that may be affected during their child's hospitalization and for which they may require assistance. Questionnaires, such as "Managing My Child's Medical Needs" described in Chapter 6, may be helpful in identifying additional training needs of family caregivers. The service coordinator may also request more extensive **needs surveys** (also described In Chapter 6) from parents, which will be used later in the development of a formal IFSP. When the child's hospitalization is not expected to be prolonged, it is best to complete the IFSP procedure after the child is discharged. It may not be possible to determine the full reality of caregiving needs until the child is actually in the home, so completing the IFSP once the child is at home may prove most practical. For infants for whom prolonged hospitalization is expected, the formal IFSP may best be completed while the child is still in the hospital and then revised after discharge.

During the child's hospitalization, it is helpful for intervention to begin as soon as possible. Therefore, an interim plan that targets both the needs of the family and those of the infant during the hospitalization should be developed immediately. Interviews with the family caregivers may be adequate to ascertain what aspects of family functioning need support during hospitalization. These may include needs relating to sibling care, transportation, more specific training, or counseling needs. The family must then specify the relative importance of these needs and determine the order in which they should be addressed.

The interim plan needs to be flexible to assess and address family needs as they evolve during hospitalization. Needs for support may fluctuate with the child's health status. The "roller-coaster" analogy to the PICU course is one frequently expressed by families. When infants take downturns, the family may need more intensive emotional support.

DEVELOPMENT OF THE INPATIENT INTERVENTION PLAN

Following a formal evaluation of child and family needs, an **intervention plan** should be devised to identify the specific goals to be addressed during the infant's hospitalization. The goals should be mutually agreed upon by both the family and the staff. They may range anywhere from interests in feeding issues to helping a sibling adjust to the hospitalization. Often, the family's stated needs and priorities for a child may be related less to developmental issues than to medical ones. In this case, it is important not only to respect the family's priorities but also to initiate some discussion around the infant's developmental status and what strategies are appropriate to support development during hospitalization. *Setting developmental goals can often help to shift some of the focus away from strictly medical issues and can help parents to view the infant in a more holistic manner.*

Service Coordination

An assigned service coordinator plays an important role in implementation of the intervention plan. Using a primary service coordination system when providing early intervention services to hospitalized infants can be extremely advantageous for both family and staff (Davis and Steel, 1991). Throughout the course of a hospitalization, the service coordinator acts as a liaison between the family and other professional hospital staff. This individual is often the "touchstone" for families through an extended period of the child's illness both in and out of the hospital. A full discussion of the theory and practice underlying service coordination and functions of the service coordinator is offered in Chapter 6.

The service coordinator is responsible for coordinating the infant's **inpatient developmental intervention plan.** The service coordinator consults with the other team members when a child is enrolled in services or when the child is rehospitalized. At that time, a decision should be made as to how assessment of the child will proceed. The service coordinator then becomes responsible for:

- Coordinating the assessment with the family and team
- Receiving appropriate activity suggestions from other team members
- Posting activity suggestions by the infant's bed.

The service coordinator will find it helpful to alert medical caregivers to the infant's involvement in early intervention services. A note to this effect along with a summary of the infant's current developmental status should be placed in the medical chart, so that medical professionals working with the infant are aware of this aspect of the child. An **identifying sticker** that is recognized by hospital staff might be affixed to posted plans to remind them of the child's involvement in an intervention plan. These may be attached to the infant's medical chart as well as to the crib.

Communication

An "introduction" of the some of the personal characteristics of the infant and family to medical caregivers and therapists on the floor helps make the admission of the child to the inpatient service easier on both the family and staff. An **information**

sheet, detailing the infant's abilities, preferred activities and toys, favorite foods and feeding methods, and even the child's nickname, helps to individualize the infant or toddler. The parents' phone numbers, work schedules, and typical visiting hours are also very helpful information for the staff. A model fact sheet, "All About Me," is seen in Figure E. This can easily be posted on the infant's bed or room door. It is nice to personalize the child by providing photographs of the infant herself and perhaps another of the parents and siblings.

Figure E

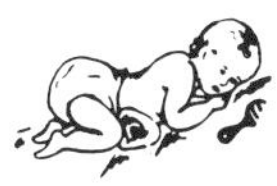

ALL ABOUT ME

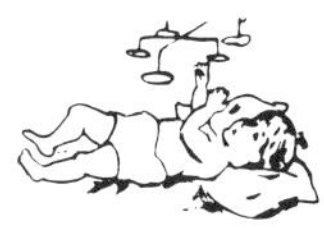

NAME:________________ PARENTS NAME:________________

NICKNAME:____________

AGE:________________

MY FAVORITE TOYS ARE:________________________________

I CAN DO THE FOLLOWING:______________________________

I USE THE FOLLOWING WORDS:___________________________

I EAT BY:____

MY USUAL NAPTIME IS:_________________________
BEDTIME IS:_________________________

I SLEEP WITH:____

MY FAVORITE GAMES ARE:_______________________________

PREFERRED POSITIONS ARE:_____________________________

SPECIAL CONSIDERATIONS:______________________________

MY PARENTS CAN BE REACHED-
DAY:________________
EVENING:________________

The service coordinator should get an idea of how long the baby will be hospitalized. The admitting note in the medical chart usually outlines the infant's status, symptoms, assessment, and proposed medical care plan. Parents, nurses, and information from patient rounds will also help to identify the expectations of the hospitalization.

If an infant will only be an inpatient for a short time (one to three days), the primary focus of the developmental team should be to provide family support, appropriate activity for the infant, and consultation to other hospital staff as needed. In a situation in which a longer hospitalization is anticipated, the **full developmental care plan** resulting from the assessment should be retained by the infant's bed. A shorter **posted care plan** should specify optimal positioning for the infant, appropriate developmental activities, and psychosocial considerations in a weekly plan. (See Figure F.) Photos taken with an instant camera help illustrate specific suggestions and may be attached to each activity sheet.

Figure F

This week I'm working on......

1) "keeping my hands together in the middle."

2) "learning to imitate simple gestures."
Encourage me to clap my hands, pat my knees, bang, or rub my fingers on a surface. Remember to do actions I can see myself do.

3) "using my memory."
Throw a washcloth or an edge of my blanket over my favorite toy, my tape recorder, or my bottle. Help me learn to search for and find it. Start by covering half of it and eventually the whole thing!

4) "helping with dressing."
Encourage me to extend my arms and legs when dressing. Let me pull off my socks.

5) "learning to make things move."
Please place my toy bar in bed with me when I am awake and alert. Position me in an infant seat or in my inner tube (see picture). Let the toys hang near enough my hands so that I can touch them.

6) "learning my name." Please call me by name when you care for me. See if I respond to my name.

7) "holding different textures and reaching for different sized objects."
When bathing me, please pull out the toys in my mesh bag (They are all waterproof). They require me to use different grasp patterns to hold them and also all have a different feel to them.

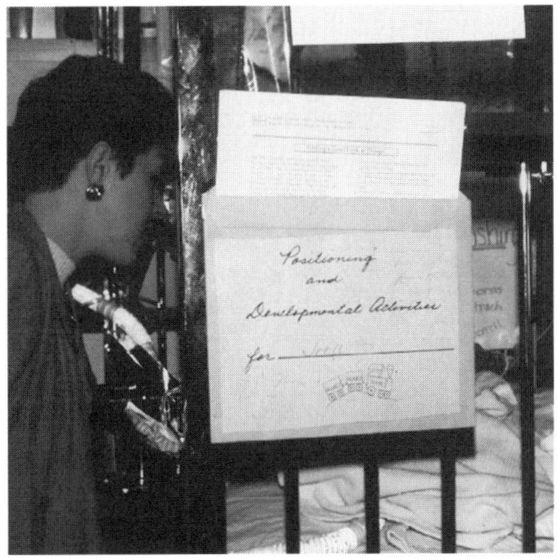

Facilitation of a **normalized routine** is an important part of each child's developmental care plan. The infant's caregiving needs, feeding schedule, and preferred sleep schedule should be discussed with the parents and nursing staff. A proposed daily routine can then be devised and assimilated into the infant's nursing care plan. In addition to the above, this daily "schedule" should include times for play, the planned therapy sessions, and specific activities, such as "music time" or "floor play". A posted daily schedule (Figure G) will familiarize everyone to the routine. It is important to allow for flexibility and to maintain a realistic sense of the infant's capabilities and stamina. Providing a daily routine can help the infant to establish anticipation of events throughout his day. The nursing staff may also find it a helpful structure to follow in planning caregiving tasks.

Figure G
Clarence's Day

7:00 - 8:00 Wake, vital signs
8:00 - 8:30 Breakfast (I eat best using a red preemie nipple.)
8:45 - 9:15 Caregiving/Bath time
(On weekends, please wait and let my mother bathe me.)
9:15 - 10:00 Physical therapy (M, W, F)
Music time (Tues, Th)
10:00 - 10:30 Quiet time in swing or infant seat with toys
10:30 - 10:45 Morning snack
10:45 - 11:45 A.M. Nap (If the unit is noisy and busy, please "drape" my crib.)
12:00 - 12:15 Caregiving, vital signs
12:15 - 1:00 Lunch (When spoon-feeding, please use the yellow tipped spoon!)
1:00 - 1:45 Early Intervention (M, W, F)
Speech therapy (Tues, Th)
1:45 - 3:00 P.M. Nap
3:00 - 4:00 **Safe Time! No procedures during this time!!**
Tues, Fri Baby Hour in the Playroom
Mon, Wed, Th Floor Play on mat or playpen with a friend.
4:00 - 4:30 Afternoon snack, caregiving
5:30 - 6:00 Mom and Dad come!
6:00 - 6:45 Dinner (If Mom and Dad are here they will feed me.)
7:00 - 7:30 Quiet time. Rocking and holding.
8:00 Bedtime

Suggested procedural guidelines for establishing an intervention plan during hospitalization are provided in Table 5.

Table 5
Procedural Steps for Implementing Intervention Program Activities for Each Child

Step	Activities
1. Identification of child as receiving early intervention services	- project sticker in chart, on bed
2. Introduction of child and family to the unit staff	- "All About Me" - photographs of child and family - summary of child's current abilities and skills
3. Identification of appropriate positioning	- photos - position stickers - activity sheet
4. Identification of appropriate developmental activities	- photos - developmental activity sheet - "This Week I'm Working on"
5. Facilitation of normalized routine	- posted daily routine/schedule
6. Facilitation of normalized environment	- toys from home - blankets, quilts - dress infant in own clothing - Baby group
7. Communication among family, intervention professionals, and medical/nursing staff	- communication book - rounds - direct consultation - medical charts
8. Continuity of care between hospital and home	- communication with community early intervention programs - home visits - phone contact - clinic visits

REHOSPITALIZATION

Direct contact by the service coordinator with the parents should be attempted as soon as possible whenever the child is rehospitalized. Hearing from a familiar hospital staff member may help to reassure the parents at a time of emotional stress. Some professionals may wish to provide families with their home phone numbers so they may be contacted in the event of an evening or weekend admission. This is often helpful to families as the medical staff may be unfamiliar, especially during these off-peak hours. Service coordinators need to maintain flexibility to best meet the needs of the child and family, particularly during a crisis period.

When the family is known to the PICU staff, a developmental plan can usually be implemented fairly quickly. Updating the current goals of the child's home-based or center-based intervention plan will be necessary. The goals may need to be modified in consideration of the child's acute illness. Direct contact between the service coordinator and the community-based interventionist will be helpful in providing continuity in programming. Formal developmental assessment may not be needed at this time if the hospital intervention team knows the child. However, evaluation of the impact of the current illness on developmental levels will be needed. It may also be helpful to include the previous developmental assessment in the medical chart so that medical caregivers are familiar with the child's abilities. A developmental plan with specific activity goals should be posted at the bedside.

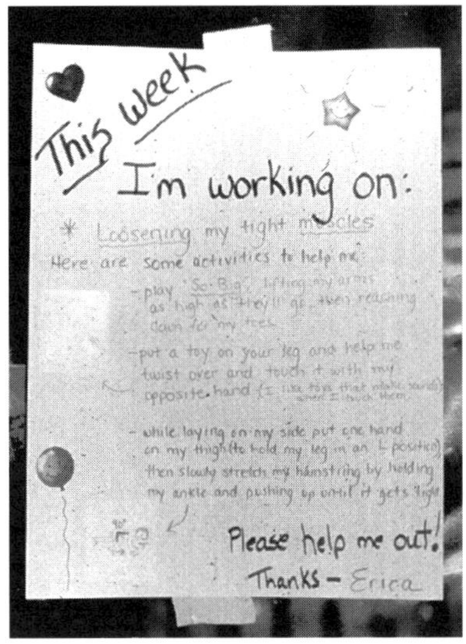

INTERVENTION STRATEGIES

ROLE OF THE INFANT DEVELOPMENT SPECIALIST

The infant development specialist on the PICU assumes, as a primary responsibility, the infant's developmental and psychological well-being during hospitalization.

Maintaining developmental goals during hospitalization is not always easy because the hospital staff's focus is on enhancing medical stability in the infant and promoting discharge. Unfortunately, not only are the child's developmental needs often a low priority, but also the very nature of the hospital experience typically slows or impedes the progression of developmental skills. Hospital staff who are aware of the potential *negative impact of hospitalization on development* may be able to make adjustments that reduce some of the deleterious effects. The following table lists some of the negative influences of hospitalization and its subsequent effect upon development that might be brought to the attention of the nursing and developmental staff (Table 6.)

The infant development specialist establishes appropriate developmental activities for the infant. Overall goals for the infant should include:

- Maintenance of existing skills
- Mastery of new skills
- Play and interaction with toys and people
- Personality development
- Self-help skills
- Prevention of emotional depression
- Prevention of regression of developmental skills

Intervention strategies for the individual infant are most helpful when developed with awareness of particular guidelines and expectations with respect to how infants

Table 6
Negative Effects of Hospitalization

- Hospitalization separates a baby from her family unit which is the optimal arena for growth and learning.

- Negative psychosocial experiences during hospitalization make an impact on the infant's desire and motivation for play and learning.

- The lack of a consistent routine and a consistent caregiver makes it difficult for an infant to have positive anticipation of events in her day.

- Physical restrictions placed on a hospitalized infant by crib, I.V.s, feeding pumps, etc. limit potential for exploration and movement.

- Pain and discomfort from illness and medical procedures often cause an infant to become lethargic, passive, and unresponsive to stimulation. It will also tend to make an infant mistrustful of people and the environment.
- Any of the above factors can induce regression of existing skills by the infant and/or retar dation of further development.

(Vessey et al., 1991)

will learn best in a hospital setting. They include the following:

- Infants learn best in an environment where they feel safe and trusting of people and events.
- Infants learn best in the context of their family.
- Infants learn from unique and novel stimulation and experiences.
- Infants build new developmental skills cumulatively based on those already acquired.
- Infants with special needs are often more passive and display less spontaneity and active exploration in their play.
- Infants learn by repeating learning activities often and practicing already acquired skills.
- Infants are most open to learning when they are alert, interested, and feeling good.
- Play is a necessary experience for acquiring developmental skills, enhancing personality development, learning creativity and exploration, and acquiring physical abilities.
- Infants learn adaptive and social behavior though normal opportunities for interaction with objects, peers, and adults.

(Wolfer et al., 1989)

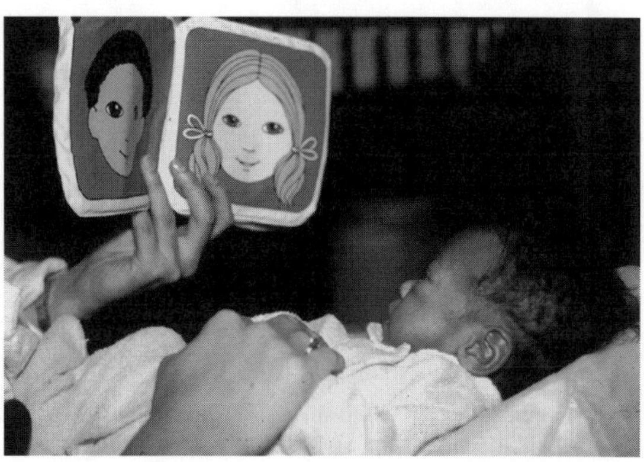

In addition to posted activities and developmental suggestions to family and staff, regular **hands-on intervention** sessions should be scheduled with the infant. If possible, the infant should be scheduled for one-on-one intervention two to three times per week. Intervention sessions should be targeted to last approximately 30 to 45 minutes, depending on the infant's alertness and stability. Intervention should be scheduled so as not to conflict with caregiving times, preferably between feedings, after naps, and apart from any medical procedures. Optimally, intervention would be most effective if it could be done in a playroom or setting away from medical surroundings. Unfortunately, this is rarely possible, and intervention must, in most cases, be conducted with the child in bed or in his hospital room.

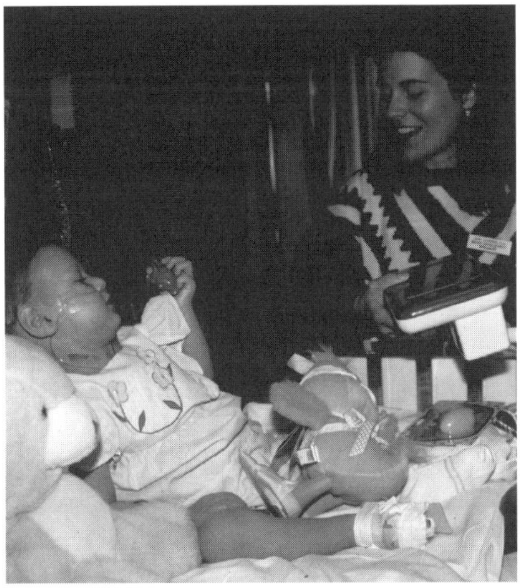

It may be helpful for the infant if intervention is scheduled at times when parents are working or not able to be present at the hospital so the infant will have some positive interaction during that time of separation. However, some sessions should be scheduled when the parents can be present, so there may be modeling and feedback around intervention techniques.

Interventionists must remain flexible at all times when they plan developmental sessions with a child. Helping nurses feed, change or clothe an infant may be necessary to get a child ready for the intervention session. This may also enhance the nursing staff's view of the interventionist's commitment. Flexibility is also necessary when it is apparent a child is not well enough to participate in the planned activity.

TOYS AND ACTIVITIES

The infant specialist will find consultation from the physical therapist of great importance when beginning work with a *very young infant or a very medically compromised child.* This is because it may be necessary to keep the handling of the child to a minimum; therefore, proper positioning of the infant to maximize sensory, physical, and interpersonal contact with the environment becomes essential. In activities, the focus will be on enhancing the child's:

- Autonomic regulation
- Visual skills
- Auditory attention
- Integration of tactile stimulation

For *older infants*, developmental activities can incorporate the following areas of conceptual development:

<u>Cause and effect</u>

- Repeatedly knocking down an object to have the adult right it
- Pulling a cord attached to an object to secure it
- Ringing a bell or shaking a rattle to hear the sound

<u>Object permanence</u>

- Dropping an object off a tray surface and searching for it visually
- Playing variations of peek-a-boo
- Hiding and uncovering an object with a cloth

<u>Imitation</u>

- Echoing the sounds an infant makes and getting her to repeat the sounds again
- Demonstrating an activity, such as patting a toy, and encouraging the child to do the same
- Singing songs or rhymes with finger plays to get the child to participate

<u>Language development</u>

- Naming objects in the environment and bringing the child's attention to them
- Leading the child through a response to a request, such as "clap hands"
- Encouraging the child to make eye contact when spoken to

The interventionist should be alert to any *signs of preference* by the child for particular toys or materials. The child may demonstrate this when he gives repeated eye gaze to a specific toy or laughs in response to the activity. By responding to the child's preference, the interventionist provides the child with the feeling that he has some control over his environment.

The infant specialist must be especially alert to *signs of fatigue or frustration* in the child. Activities must be modulated or discontinued for that session if the following behaviors are observed:

- Color changes such as paleness or blue pallor (sometimes observed best in the lip area)
- Increased respiration rate
- Slowing of the heartbeat
- Decrease in postural stability
- Marked irritability
- Oxygen saturation rate in an undesirable range
- Gaze aversion or "tuning out"

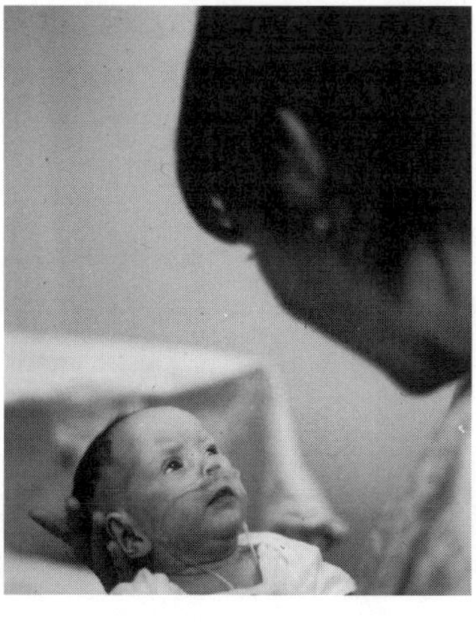

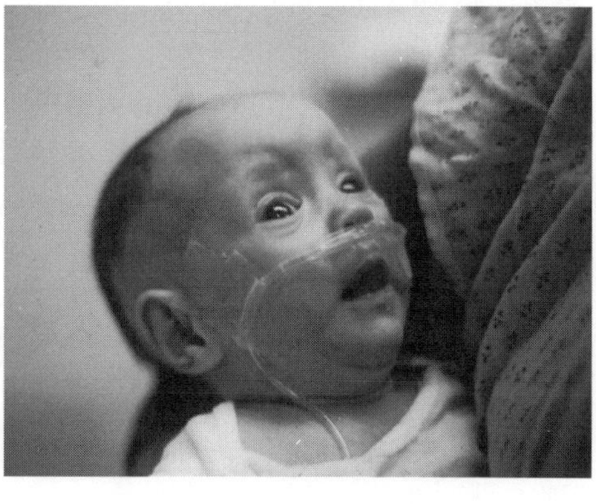

The child's nurse is the best resource for alerting the interventionist as to warning signs or monitor values that suggest the infant is experiencing stress. Guidelines as to what signs to be alert to should be determined at the beginning of the intervention plan. These may be modified, depending on the child's medical status.

Toys selected for use in intervention sessions should have the following characteristics:

- Lightweight, easily grasped
- Not easily broken
- Washable, able to be disinfected
- Multisensory (touch and sound) when possible

It is useful to have some toys affixed to the crib and others at ready access. It is important, however, that these do not obstruct access to the infant for caregiving needs. Select or adapt toys with an eye towards maintaining flexibility in their use. The following suggestions for toy selection might be considered:

- Mobiles - should be of the "screw on" variety so that they can quickly and easily be removed from the bedrail. Mobiles should be positioned with regard to the infant's vantage point.
- Play gyms - are perfect for use with this population. They are easily placed in a standard-sized hospital crib and can be stored underneath the bed without being dismantled. The optimal placement for an infant is in an infant seat with the gym in easy reaching or gazing distance. For a child who is unable to reach purposefully, a loose piece of ribbon can be tied between the dangling objects and the infant's wrist. Any random movement of the hand or arm will then activate the toys.
- Crib mirrors - should be available for each infant's crib. These are easily screwed onto the inside bars, however, they may interfere with the lowering of the crib rail. Mirrors should be placed on the side of the bed less accessed by medical staff.
- Velcro™ strips - long strips of Velcro can be attached to the top inside of covered cribs. Lightweight pompons and rattles tied to a piece of cloth ribbon with opposing Velcro can

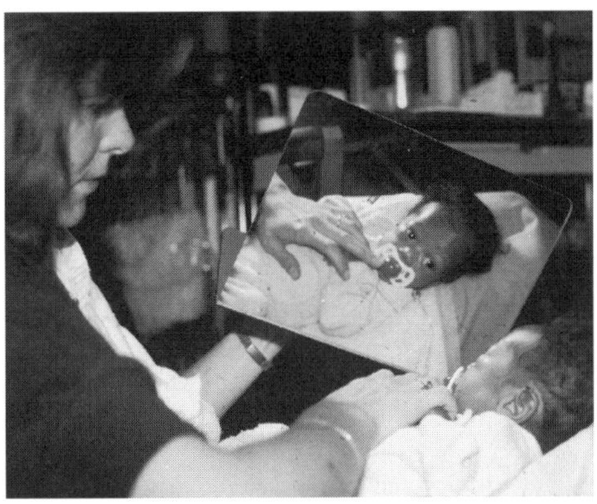

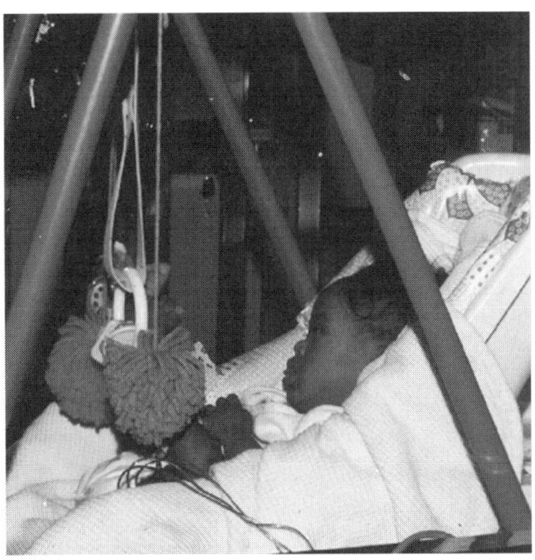

then be hung from the ceiling of the crib and can easily be detached and changed.

- Pictures/photographs - can be covered with clear contact paper and taped anywhere in the crib. Large, bright pictures taken from magazines or old calendars make excellent visual stimulation. These are also excellent for a child under an oxygen tent who has little opportunity for play. They are easily taped and removed from the top or side of the clear plastic of the tent.

- Some toys, such as a music box or tape recorder, can be modified with an adaptive switch so that an infant can receive positive feedback through even a light touch with a hand or foot. This is particularly good for motor-impaired infants. Voice-activated toys may also be appropriate, although they should be checked for level of difficulty.

An additional list of toy suggestions and intervention strategies is provided in Tables 7 and 8.

Table 7
Toys by Age Levels

0-4 Months
small, lightweight rattles with thin handles & gentle noises
crib mirror
roly-poly chime toys
black/white patterned pictures and toys
mobiles
music boxes
teething rings
soft stuffed animals
crib gyms
bells

4-8 Months
rattles
suction cup rattles
wind-up toys
teething ring
activity boards
squeak toys
ankle rattles
toys near my feet to kick
music box
crib mirror
plastic keys
plastic measuring spoons

8-12 Months
picture books
activity boards
pop-up boxes
nesting cups
small blocks
jack-in-the-box
bubbles
wooden spoons and sauce pan with lid
ring stacker
music
pop beads

12-18 Months
pull & push toys
blocks
nesting cups
large pegs & pegboard
shape sorters
books
toy telephone
2-4 piece puzzles
See-n-Say
baby doll
doll bottle & blanket
crayons & paper
toy musical instruments
nursery rhyme tapes & records

18-24 Months
Play-Doh™
water colors, finger paints
sandbox
play tools
simple story books
small wagon or grocery cart
empty food containers
3-5 piece puzzles
dress-up clothes
small people, cars, animals
building blocks
large Lego™ blocks

Table 8
Equipment & Techniques for Facilitating Activities in the PICU

1) Developmentally Appropriate Toys
- toy cabinet-storage area in playroom
- best organized by type of activity:
  - toys for reaching & grasping
  - visually stimulating toys
  - music

2) Opportunity for floor play
- small portable mats to be kept under each child's bed
- can be used with a child on IVs

3) Adaptive Equipment
- storage area on PICU for:
  - feeder seats
  - infant seats
  - prone standers
  - wedge
  - rolls
  - therapy balls

4) Opportunity for structured tabletop activities
- wooden blocks
- "box desks" covered with contact paper

5) Crib Toys
- port-a-gyms
- crib mirrors
- Velcro™ stripping strung across bed with toys attached *(watch for safety)*

6) Access/storage of toys in child's room
- drawstring mesh laundry bag attached to crib bar
- small empty diaper box at end of bed
- inverted "box desk"

7) Relaxation activities
- crib hammocks
- infant swings
- massage lotion
- tapes of nursery rhymes, parents' and sibling' voices

8) Organization of toys and equipment return
- "Toy Return" box on unit where toys can be dropped for cleaning and storage
- toys labeled and washed regularly

PSYCHOSOCIAL DEVELOPMENT

Many factors make a hospitalization overstimulating and stressful to an infant. The PICU is a place where infants experience unfamiliar clothes, strange people and toys, and different feeding and sleeping arrangements. There are many restrictions that affect play, motor activity, and exploratory behaviors. In addition, painful procedures and separation from family work against the infant's ability to trust her environment, one of infancy's well-recognized developmental tasks. Children below the age of five are most vulnerable because they are not yet able to understand verbal explanations of what is happening to them or to express fears.

Appropriate psychosocial care should be designed to include the following considerations:

- Facilitation or maintenance of parent/infant attachment
- Interaction with siblings
- Continuity of care by staff who are specially trained in the unique developmental needs of children and families
- Encouragement of normal growth and development
- Opportunities for pleasurable stimulation such as talking, stroking, and holding
- Enhancement or maintenance of self-help skills
- Encouragement of individual personality characteristics

(Wolfer et al, 1989)

An infant's social responsiveness provides important reinforcement for parents. Effects of medications or the illness itself may reduce the infant's social responsivity or produce irritability. This, in turn, provides negative feedback to parents and may diminish their enthusiasm in nurturing the infant. Repeated hospitalization interrupts the flow of family development and may impede the sense of parental competence (Perrin and Gerrity, 1984). Support of the family with respect to these issues is an integral part of the emotional care of the infant.

Adequate **physical interaction and bonding** may be difficult for parents if their infant is attached by tubes and wires to high tech medical equipment. Some parents may be afraid and reluctant to hold their child. The staff should be supportive and attempt to facilitate parental competence and confidence in handling their infant. It is important to explain the medical equipment to parents and reduce the mystique by allowing them to touch the various tubes and buttons. Providing the parents with knowledge about the function of the machinery will give them a greater understanding of their infant's course of treatment and daily status. Before a parent holds a child attached to equipment, proper handling techniques should be demonstrated so that parents can feel sure that both they and their infant will be comfortable. Initially, staff should be present to assist by putting the baby into the parents' arms and providing them with position suggestions and feedback on their technique.

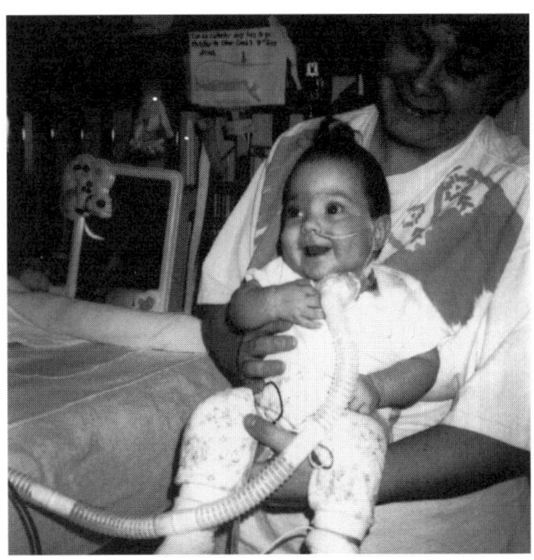

Making the infant's hospital environment seem more *familiar* to him should be a consideration. Parents should be encouraged to bring in familiar belongings from home labeled with the child's name. These might include toys, blankets, pillows, clothes and room decorations that may help increase the infant's sense of security. The nursing staff should be encouraged to dress the infant in his own clothes when appropriate. A sign attached to the bed saying, "Please dress me in my cutest outfit" may be a friendly reminder to the staff.

Parents should be encouraged to advocate for their baby in all areas of caregiving. For example, they may want to ask the staff not to bathe the baby in the morning so they can do it when they arrive in the afternoon. Designating the use of a specific spoon or bottle that belongs to the infant may help to improve feeding and can be comforting and reassuring to the infant.

Building some *inviolate quiet time* into the infant's daily routine is an important consideration. During a prolonged hospitalization, the infant will likely become aware of the patterns in her day and may develop the ability to relax during this quiet period. Earmarking this time by playing a specific tape or singing a particular song every day will help identify this **"safe time"** for the infant. To assure consistency, these strategies will need to be outlined in the infant's care plan or daily schedule, so that nursing staff are aware of and can help to implement this routine.

Peer Interaction

It is often observed that children can be wonderful medicine for one another. Whenever possible, attempts should be made to *facilitate social interaction* among infants and toddlers on the PICU. This may be accomplished by positioning two infants side by side in swings, infant seats, or a playpen, or allowing several infants to play together on a floor mat. For an infant who is crib-bound, it may involve holding another baby up to the side of the crib so the two can look and possibly reach out to one another. Of course, precaution must always be taken with respect to medical stability and the possible spread of infection. Checking with the nursing staff is essential before bringing any children together.

If the PICU has a playroom, a time can be set for infants to be taken there one or more times a week for a group session. The infant development specialist must collaborate with the nursing staff and physicians to identify infants who are capable of participating. Infants who are stable enough to participate may be brought to the playroom on a tele-monitoring system that allows them to be detached from their room monitors. This group intervention time should be written into their daily routine so the nursing staff will be sure that the children are fed and rested before "Baby Hour" begins. If the playroom is equipped with an electrical outlet panel and oxygen support hook-ups, infants on I.V.s, feeding pumps, nasal cannulas, and infusion pumps will all be able to participate in the group. A call button and telephone should be available in the event that medical staff need to be summoned at any time.

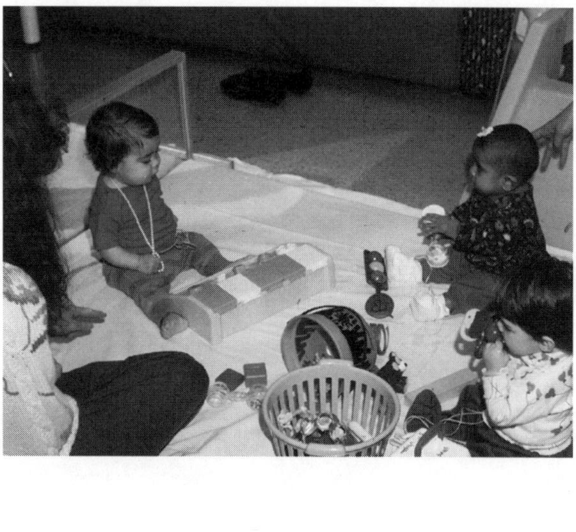

A **play group** of this nature allows infants to spend some quality time in a more normalized social environment and helps provide a focus other than medical and illness-related issues. The play environment provides enjoyment to both the infant and parent, and medical staff are also pleased at seeing the infant benefit from stimulation and peer interaction. Parents may get ideas about how to encourage peer interaction when the child returns home. General social, sensory, motor, and cognitive intervention activities should be planned for each hour. Toymaking activities may be made available for parents who are interested (See Table 9.). A one-to-one (or at most, one-to-two) staff and parent ratio is probably necessary. Depending on the available hospital staff, support staff for the group may be drawn from graduate interns, child-life specialists, physical or occupational therapists, or older pediatric patients on the unit with adequate maturity and interest. This "big brother/big sister" approach can be very socially and emotionally beneficial to both older and younger patients.

Table 9
Suggestions for Toymaking

Article	Necessary Materials
- yarn pompon ball (for tracking, batting, and tactile experience)	pom-pon makers available at craft stores for under $5; use bright colored, synthetic yarn
- wrist/ankle rattles	1/2 " wide elastic material; jingle bell; thread
- rattles	cigar tubes, prescription bottles, film canisters: fill with beans, unpopped popcorn. cover with contact paper or fabric. toilet paper rolls: fill, seal at end with paper or cardboard, cover with contact paper.
- mobiles	coat hangers with toys suspended. Can be hooked over Velcro™ stripping in crib. Sharp hook end should be taped. Wooden needlework rings hung with toys attached .
- eye-catchers	paper plates with black and white design; magazine photos; family photos covered with clear contact paper; colored mylar strips; ribbons fashioned into bunches
- kick boxes	paper towel, cardboard roll, oatmeal, or salt boxes: filled, covered and hung at infant's feet
- peek-a-boo board	mirror, decorated cardboard square, or family picture: cover with fabric flap fastened at top, loose at bottom
- tactile variety objects	pot scrubber, sponges, Koosh™ balls

COLLABORATION WITH STAFF AND PARENTS

Successful early intervention services can only be ensured if there is *optimal communication and collaboration* between interventionists and the physician, nurse, and parent caregivers. It is important to develop good working relationships with all of those involved in the family's care. Maintaining a high level of visibility on the PICU itself is necessary for the intervention staff to earn trust among the medical staff. Developing a working knowledge of the unit and standard operating procedures is imperative. Keeping abreast of patients' medical status, floor admissions and discharges, and general medical knowledge about pediatric conditions will help lend credibility to the nonmedical professional.

Intervention team members should seek to become included in **patient rounds** - medical rounds, family rounds, or both. These meetings provide medical updates for each patient on the unit, covering the present course of treatment, family and developmental issues, and discharge planning. Family rounds are usually attended by nursing staff, social workers, pastoral care staff, child-life specialists, and therapists. In this forum, professionals share knowledge from each of their specialties, and the team can discuss various approaches for best meeting the needs of each child and family. The intervention team members can review the child's developmental status and pass along related suggestions to participating medical staff at rounds.

Bedside plans, activities, and schedules all help to increase awareness and communication of the infant's developmental needs. Activities should be changed regularly (once a week) to ensure variety for both the infant and staff. Direct consultation with the nursing staff concerning optimal positions or feeding strategies may be advantageous, particularly for infants with complex needs.

"**Communication books**" (blank, hard-cover journals) may be given to each family and kept by the infant's bed throughout a hospitalization. This provides a means in which interventionists, parents, and medical staff can have regular contact regarding information about the infant. Pictures, photographs, progress notes, updates, and activity suggestions can easily be exchanged by all parties. This means of communication is particularly valuable when parents are restricted in their visiting availability or are working during the day. Many parents also find this a nice keepsake.

A "**graffiti sheet**" may be placed alongside the posted activity plan to encourage the participation of the medical staff in the developmental intervention activities. The nursing/medical staff then may write short personalized comments, such as, "Mark did a great job sitting with help!" or "Susie sat for 10 seconds alone today!" This provides a means for brief input from the caregiving staff as well as a way of letting the parents know that the nursing/medical staff are also working on the developmental activities. Progress notes, placed in the medical chart, provide a more comprehensive description of the intervention for the staff and should be updated regularly.

In-service programs are beneficial to help the medical/nursing staff keep abreast of family and developmental issues in pediatric health care. Early intervention team members can offer to lead discussions around issues such as optimal positioning and handling, feeding techniques, communication with family members, involving siblings, and general developmental needs of the hospitalized infant. Usually these issues may be coordinated through the unit's clinical nurse educator. Flexibility may be necessary to access staff between shift changes or at monthly unit staff meetings, which will often be before or after regular working hours.

It is important to maintain an appropriate understanding of each professional's role and involvement with the infant. The nursing staff should not be expected to act as interventionists. Developmental suggestions targeted towards the nursing staff should be caregiving related (feeding, positioning, social interaction), so that they are easily incorporated into the nurse's already committed time with the infant. Parents, too, should be encouraged to maintain their role as parents, not as full-time interventionists. It is easy to place unrealistic expectations on both the parents and staff. *Encouraging awareness of developmental needs, appreciation of the early intervention philosophy, and importance of family involvement should be the primary goals in this regard.*

REFINEMENT OF INTERVENTION GOALS

When an infant is hospitalized for a prolonged period, the developmental care plan should be updated on a monthly basis. **Weekly team staffings** provide a regular forum in which the infant's status and progress can be discussed and program modifications added. Parents should be actively involved in helping to establish ongoing goals for their infant. Any changes in plans should be communicated to nursing caregivers. New photos and listed activities should reflect changes in the developmental plan.

Intervention staff must be aware that program modification can go in one of two directions. Goals may be set at more advanced development levels as the child matures and becomes more medically stable. It is often the case, however, that chronically ill children will suffer medical setbacks so that developmental goals will need to be scaled down for a time.

When a child is readmitted onto the PICU after some length of time at home, intervention goals will need to be reviewed and updated. The IFSP itself should also be modified as needed to meet the family's changing needs. The infant may have progressed both medically and developmentally so that previous goals are no longer appropriate. An informal meeting between service coordinator, family, relevant team members, and nursing staff should be held to identify these issues. Parents may be asked to describe the infant's recent activities and behaviors at home. In addition, information from community early intervention programs and therapists should be obtained so that consistency is maintained in intervention approaches. This information may then be incorporated into a developmental care plan as on previous or initial admissions. The bedside developmental curriculum plan should be updated by the various team members, who will then establish appropriate developmental activities for each domain of development.

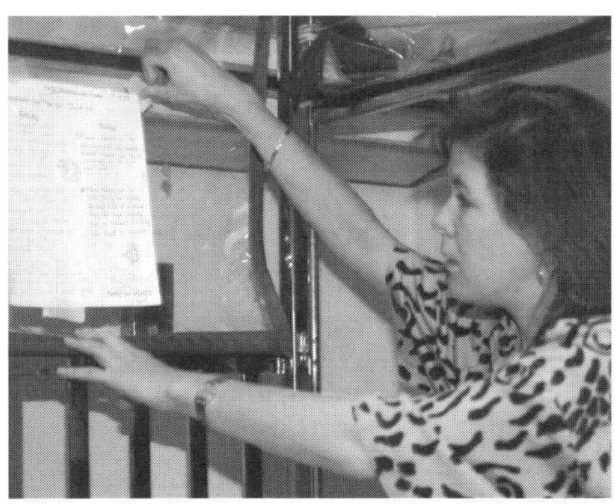

PHYSICAL THERAPY INTERVENTION IN THE PICU

Like the infant specialist, the physical therapist also provides an important direct service role for infants in the PICU. The most essential part of physical therapy is to promote movement. Through movement children learn motor skills and are able to explore their environment. Children in the PICU are often deprived of much of the spontaneous movement a healthy child experiences. Therefore, the physical therapist's role in the PICU is to promote motor learning to the extent possible by planned motor strategies and adaptation of the environment. While this discussion will refer specifically to physical therapy, it is important to be aware that there is considerable overlap with **occupational therapy**, and in most instances, these strategies can be used by either discipline.

Physical therapy intervention in the PICU involves assessment, intervention, parent education, and staff education. In order to effectively and safely carry out the physical therapy role in this environment, the therapist must have the following skills:

1) Specific training in working with medically compromised children; the ability to interpret information from physiological monitors and to understand the function of medical equipment in relationship to the patients' medical needs
2) A working knowledge of normal development
3) An appreciation for developmental patterns characteristic of chronically ill children.

Intervention begins with identifying the *neuromotor problems* of the infant within the framework of his medical condition. Table 10 provides a list of neuromotor problems commonly experienced by the infants. Once specific problem areas are targeted by the therapist, the treatment plan in respect to neuromotor goals is formulated. In the following discussion, treatment approaches that address common neuromotor

Table 10
Common Neuromotor Problems of Chronically Ill Infants

- Hypotonia
- Hypertonia
- Poor head control
- Developmental delay
- Oral-Motor deficits
- Abnormal postures
    - hyperextension of the neck
    - full body arching
    - surrender position
    - elevated and retracted shoulders
    - frog leg position
- Poor midline skills
- Lack of flexor activity
- Tactile defensiveness
- Loss of previously acquired motor skills
- Poor endurance
- Lack of age appropriate weight-bearing skills
- Poor modulation in response to stimuli
- Musculoskeletal deformity
- Sensory deficits
- Lack of weight-shifting ability

problems encountered in chronically ill infants and young children will be reviewed. These goals must be integrated into goals set for cognitive, language, and psychosocial development so there is consistency in the plan.

Positioning

Positioning is an essential component of physical therapy. Positioning is often the only type of PT intervention that children can tolerate when they are extremely ill or very immature. Proper positioning improves muscle tone, promotes good postural alignment, facilitates developmental skills, provides the child with a different view of the environment, and prevents skin breakdown. As used in this context, "good postural alignment" refers to a symmetrical position which facilitates motor function. The therapeutic positions most frequently used include side-lying, prone, supine, sitting, and standing.

Side-lying is beneficial in that it:

- Promotes midline skills
- Facilitates good muscle tone
- Encourages good shoulder alignment and reaching
- Promotes gastric emptying when positioned on the right side

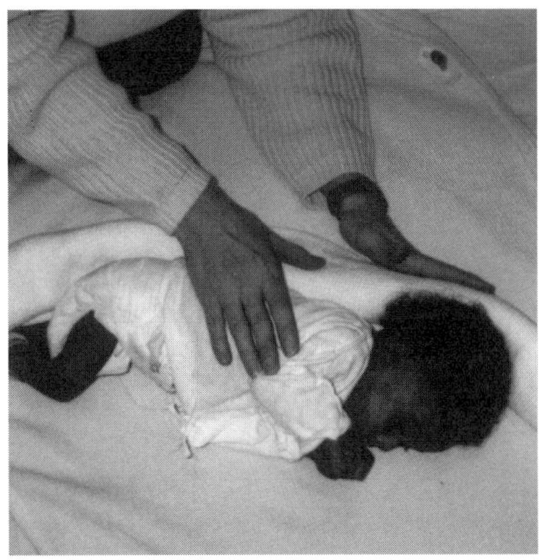

A child placed in side-lying should be well supported. *Blanket rolls* should be placed behind the child to maintain the position. A roll may also be placed *between the legs* to promote natural hip alignment and/or to limit pressure between the legs. An older child may need a small pillow placed *under the head* to maintain central alignment of the head, neck, and shoulder girdle. The young infant should be provided something to hold in order to promote good shoulder positioning and midline skill development.

The older child should have a toy or activity placed in front of him, so that he can play using his hands together. While commercial side-lyers are available, if the child can be maintained with blanket rolls, this is usually more comfortable and also more economical.

The **prone position** may be difficult for some infants to tolerate if they lack experience in this position, or have in place endotracheal tubes, gastrostomy tubes, or other medical lines. However, prone placement is a good position for these infants because it promotes:

- Flexion
- Head control
- Extension throughout the body
- Good muscle tone
- Weight-bearing through the shoulders and hips

The prone position can be maintained with rolled blankets placed *along the child's sides and under the chest.* If the infant is very young, a roll may be placed under the hips. With older children, a roll *under the hips* is not needed, as lengthening of the hip flexors and abductors in prone is a normal part of development.

Supine is the position in which most hospitalized older infants and children spend the majority of their time. From a therapeutic motor standpoint, it is generally *not the position of choice* because it encourages abnormal extension, shoulder retraction and "frog" positioning of the lower extremities. However, since the supine position makes quick access for medical interventions possible, it is regarded as a "safe" position by nursing staff and is perhaps overused. On the positive side, supine is a good position in which to interact with the child.

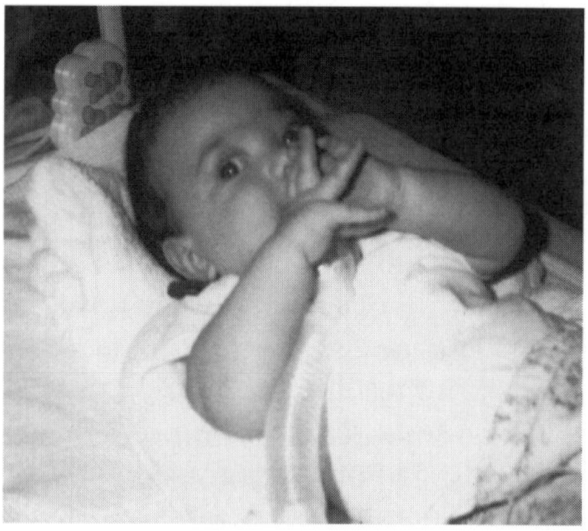

If the supine position is indicated, good postural alignment and flexion should be encouraged. *Blanket rolls* may be placed *underneath the shoulders and along the trunk* to reduce shoulder retraction and promote midline positioning of the hands. If the child cannot maintain his/her head in midline, a rolled blanket should be placed *curved around the child's head.* [see picture next] In addition, a blanket roll may be placed *under the knees* to promote flexion.

An alternative to blanket rolls for small infants is the use of a *swim ring.* The infants can be placed in the swim ring in supine. The swim ring promotes body flexion by flexing the hips and neck. Blanket rolls may be needed to fill in the gap between the shoulders and the bed to reduce stress on the neck and support the upper extremities in flexion.

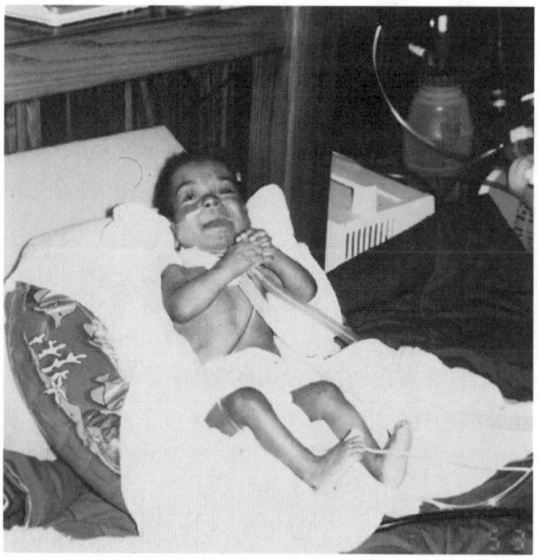

Supported **sitting** and independent sitting are important positions for the developing child. Sitting allows the child to view his world from a vertical perspective and enables the child to use his hands freely to interact with the environment. There are many ways to assist a child in maintaining a good sitting position. The seating choice depends upon the developmental level, physical size, and medical stability of the child.

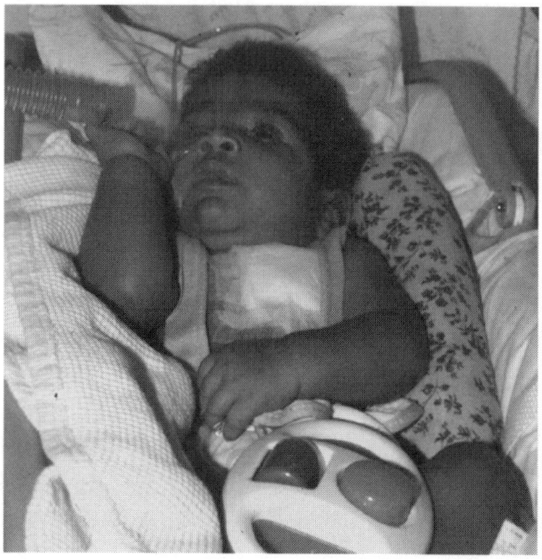

An *infant seat* may be used to provide a small, medically fragile infant with exposure to an upright position. Infant seats usually have a certain amount of adjustability in terms of the tilt in space. A fragile child, or a child who is not accustomed to sitting, should be positioned at a reclined angle.

Older and more medically stable infants can be placed in a more upright position. Blanket rolls should be placed to encourage symmetry, bring the shoulders forward, and flex the hips.

Older and/or larger infants and children can be placed in "Tumbleform™" feeder seats as an alternative to infant seats. These seats are designed to provide good postural alignment and promote flexion. These seats can be moved to adjust the amount of recline. In addition, the shoulder safety straps on the "Tumbleform™" seats provide restraint to the upper part of the body as well as to the waist. However, these straps can be a problem when a child is attached to many medical tubes or lines.

Children who have more advanced motor skills can be placed in a more upright position if they are medically stable. There are many options at this level, including toddler chairs, corner chairs, bolster chairs, and benches. The important points to remember in the use of these chairs are to:

- Encourage symmetry
- Maintain neutral alignment of the head, neck, shoulders, and hips
- Support the feet
- Ensure that all medical lines are free and untangled

Providing experience in a **standing position** is important to maintain bone density and to promote bone growth in children who developmentally approach the one-year level. Most children who achieve this level of motor development do not have to be positioned in standing because they will attempt to pull to stand in the crib or playpen. When children are sufficiently medically stable to tolerate a standing position, but are unable to stand independently due to their particular developmental problems, they may be placed in a *prone or supine stander.* This allows a child to be safely positioned in standing with good alignment and an opportunity for weight-bearing experience. The child can be positioned by a table top and encouraged to play with objects. This will increase the child's tolerance to remain in standing. Putting objects at midline and to each side will promote trunk rotation in a variety of directions and will promote development of midline and bilateral upper extremity skills.

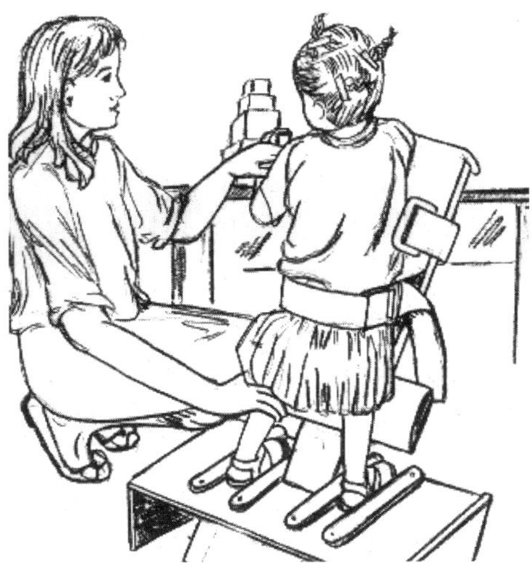

OTHER STRATEGIES

Two other strategies are used by the physical therapist in *addressing neuromotor problems* of the infant. These are **direct handling** and providing **guidance to care providers** on enhancing motor development. Direct handling sessions most often last between 30 minutes and one hour. Before a session begins, it is necessary for the therapist to read the recent progress notes in the medical chart, discuss the child's current status with her nurse, and become familiar with the child's baseline heart rate, respiration rate, and oxygen saturation level. The nurse can offer guidelines as to monitor levels that suggest the infant is being stressed.

Direct handling provides opportunities for independent, spontaneous, and assisted movement. Practice is necessary to master new movements. Therapy is essentially a time to practice these new motor skills. For instance, a therapy session may focus on improving sitting balance. The session would revolve around activities in sitting, such as reaching above the head with both hands. This activity would challenge the child's ability to maintain balance while using his chest and trunk extension to reach above his head. The therapist would support the child as needed. This activity would be practiced several times, along with other activities in this position.

Introduction of new skills is also stressed during direct handling. A new skill may be a small movement, such as a weight shift in prone on the elbows to allow the infant to reach. It may also involve a more pronounced movement, such as attaining standing from kneeling. Movement requires motor control and coordination of muscles. To further increase the child's abilities in **sitting**, activities involving reaching with weight shifting or moving into sitting from supine could be incorporated. The weight shifting and the transition from supine to sitting would be new skills expanding on the ability to maintain sitting when placed. The therapist does not perform these movements for the child, but assists the child in performing the movement herself. It may be necessary to passively move a child in order for the child to understand what is wanted, but this should always be followed with attempts to get the child to actively participate. Even though this is still an assisted movement, it is geared towards the child's achieving independent, spontaneous movement.

ADDRESSING SPECIFIC NEUROMOTOR PROBLEMS

Abnormalities in Muscle Tone

Abnormalities of muscle tone are common in this population and will be briefly explained. However, assessment of muscle tone is meaningless without assessment of functional movement patterns or skills. One must be aware that the term *muscle tone* is difficult to define (Montgomery and Connally, 1991).

One typical category of abnormal muscle tone is **hypotonia.** Hypotonia refers to low muscle tone. A child with low muscle tone is characteristically floppy and has excessive range of motion in his joints. The child typically has poor head control and shallow breathing as well (Tecklin, 1989). In addition, the child will often lock his joints when in weight-bearing positions such as prone on hands or in standing. Hypotonia in the chronically ill pediatric population may be due to a problem in the central nervous system or to extreme weakness secondary to the illness of the child.

Hypertonia represents the opposite problem in which the child shows high muscle tone. Children with hypertonia generally feel stiff. Resistance is often felt when the limbs are moved passively. Movement is difficult for these children and they show a limited variety of movement patterns. Children with hypertonicity may have hypotonia in the trunk musculature with stiffness in the upper extremities. The muscle tone increases or changes with movement or effort by the child. One of the more common postures of a chronically ill child showing hypertonicity is neck hyperextension accompanied by shoulder elevation and retraction.

The physical therapist does not address the problems of muscle tone directly, but attempts to facilitate functional movement. The goal of therapy is to increase the variety of movement patterns and to assist the child in learning new motor skills.

Encouraging Head Control

Head control refers to the ability to maintain the head in upright. The typical infant develops head control in the first few months of life by first gaining control of the neck extensors. This allows the child to lift his head and turn it when she is in prone. However, in the early weeks of life the infant cannot maintain her head in a midline position in prone or in supine due to insufficient development of the anterior neck flexors. As the child gains control of the anterior neck flexors, she is able to maintain her head erect. Good head control is established by the sixth month (Bly, 1983). The chronically ill infant is often delayed in developing control of her anterior neck flexors and therefore, has difficulty establishing adequate head control. The lack of development of the anterior neck flexors may be attributed to many things. Premature infants lack physiologic flexion that full-term infants possess at birth. Infants or children who are intubated for long periods of time are often forced into neck hyperextension on account of the mechanics of the medical equipment upon which they remain dependent. This shortens their neck extensors, making it more difficult for their anterior neck muscles to develop. Finally, children who have spent the majority of their lives on their backs by medical necessity or poor positioning have not developed the lengthened anterior musculature resulting from opportunities for prone head lifting. Central nervous system insults typical of premature status combine with some of the positioning problems described above to make the development of head control a common problem in the PICU population.

Depending upon the child's age, current ability level, and medical stability, there are a variety of ways to improve head control. With very small infants, the therapist's or parent's lap is often the best location to work on improving head control. If the child can tolerate the prone position, he can be placed with a small rolled blanket under his chest. The child can be encouraged to lift his head through the use of a toy, voice, etc. Light tapping on the neck extensors can help to encourage head lifting. The therapist may need to provide support at the shoulder girdle and humerus for stability. The child should be allowed to practice this several times, although it is important to observe skin color changes, respiration rate, heart rate, oxygen saturation rate, and behavioral cues, so that the child does not become overly fatigued.

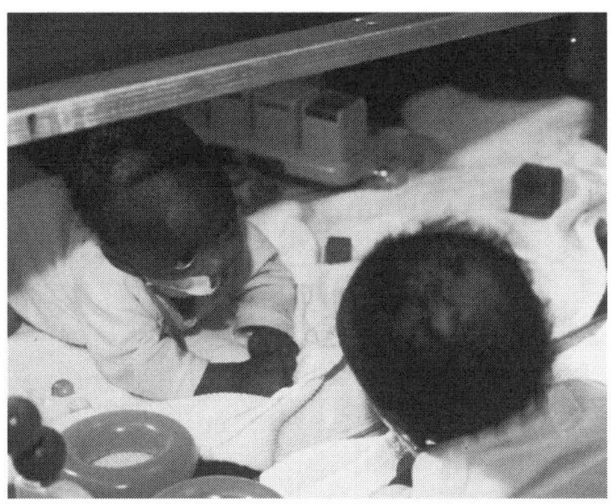

Activation of the anterior neck flexors can also be addressed in supine. If there is poor shoulder girdle and neck alignment, this should be focused on first. This is accomplished by gently bringing the shoulders down and forward. The infant's head may be placed in slight flexion using a small rolled blanket behind the neck. The therapist can then encourage chin tucking by placing an interesting toy on the infant's abdomen or gently, but firmly, tapping the chest muscles. *Tapping of the anterior part of the neck should be avoided as this is very uncomfortable and can produce an adverse reaction.* As the child becomes more adept at chin tucking, she can be gently pulled by the arms slowly to the upright position. During the movement, the infant should be given sufficient time to respond with activation of the neck flexors. Discourage the child from substituting shoulder elevation with retraction or protraction, or excessive hyperextension of the neck in lieu of activation of the neck flexors.

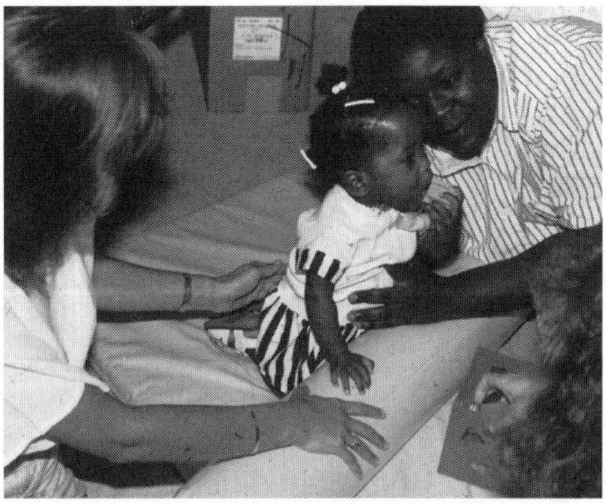

Older children with poor head control can benefit from these same activities on the bed or floor. If these children are more medically stable, there are other positions for them. A child can be placed over a bolster with her weight supported through the elbows or hands, depending upon the developmental level of the child. While in this position, the child can be encouraged to maintain the head erect. This activity can be carried out in a similar fashion by using a wedge for support. Equipment should be carefully monitored to ensure that medical tubing does not get trapped beneath the adaptive equipment.

When the child has progressed in his head control abilities, he can be placed in prone on a tilt board or ball. *The tilt board and ball should be used only after extensive instruction from a trained individual as this equipment can put the child at physical risk if not properly controlled.* While stabilizing the child at the pelvis, the surface can be tilted, allowing the child an opportunity to realign his head in a vertical position. The tilt board allows a lateral tilt, or one in the anterior-posterior direction, depending upon the position of the child on the board. Use of the ball allows movement in many planes as well as providing a more pliant surface. The therapist should at times move the surface, without warning the child, to help the child develop the use of feedback from his body in order to correct his head position. At other times the therapist should tell the child that she is going to move him, and in what direction, in order to help the child develop an anticipatory response.

Caution should be taken in the above activities when working with a child on medical technical supports. *If the child has a tracheostomy or endotracheal tube these must not be obstructed or displaced.* Children with ventriculoperitoneal shunts should not be allowed to remain in a pronounced head lag position for more than a few minutes. It is best if the child's nurse is at close call throughout the physical therapy session.

Improving Function of Flexor Musculature

The importance of the development of the flexor muscles of the body was touched on in the preceding discussion on head control. Flexion is important in performing such activities as rolling, midline skills, and reaching. Good control of flexion coupled with good control of extension is necessary to the development of upright postures. Chronically ill children typically have poor development of flexion, and therapists working in the PICU environment need to spend much of their time working on developing flexion in functional skills.

One functional way to work on the development of flexion is through **hand-to-foot play**. Supine or semi-reclined are good positions to work on hand-to-foot play. For instance, the child may be placed in supine in a swim ring as described in the section on positioning. The child is then well positioned to see his feet. Socks with bells can be placed on the child's feet and the child may be encouraged to reach for her feet. It may be helpful to assist the child by lifting her pelvis up slightly to bring her feet closer to her hands. The swim ring helps to maintain a flexed posture while the interventionist attempts to elicit active movement in flexion from the child. The semi-reclined position allows gravity to assist the body in maintaining flexion.

Hand-to-foot play may be developmentally inappropriate for the older child, but flexion can be encouraged through such games as having the child curl up in a ball while supine and pretending he is a snowball. This game or a similar one can be done on a wedge to allow gravity to assist. The functional goal should always be developmentally appropriate for the child.

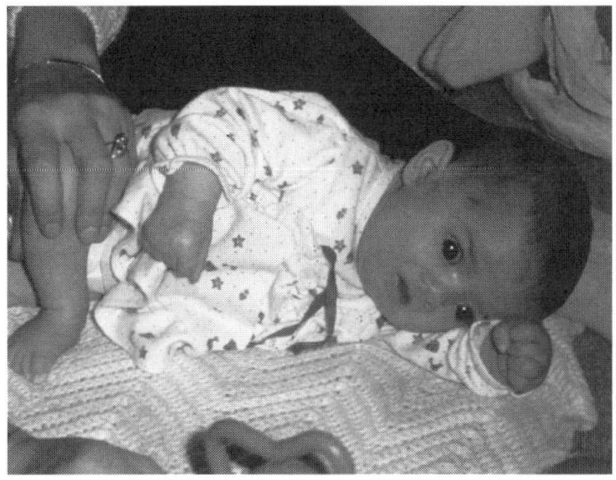

Rolling is an activity requiring activation of the flexor musculature. It is an important skill for mobility and exploring the environment. Rolling may be facilitated on the child's bed or on a floormat. The movement can be initiated at the pelvis or the shoulder girdle. It is often easier to start at the pelvis by flexing the child's leg and bringing it across the body.

The child should be given time to independently try to bring her arm and head over. If the child is unable to accomplish this, she may be assisted with support at the shoulder girdle. Another way of assisting the child to roll is to place her on a small incline, such as a wedge or slightly elevated bed. In this position, gravity again can assist the child in using her flexor muscles. Good chin tucking should be encouraged throughout the roll. While a chin tuck should be encouraged, placement of medical lines may make this difficult. To encourage movement, an environmental "lure" may be necessary. The therapist may need to try a variety of stimuli, including various toys or the therapist himself, to motivate the child.

<u>Reaching</u>

Two motor tasks that require good flexion are **reaching** and bringing **hands to midline**. Reaching is important for exploring and interacting with the environment. The development of midline skills is important for use of the two sides of the body together. The typical infant learns to bring his hands together in midline by three months and learns to swipe at an object by four months of age (Bly, 1983). These movements require good control of the anterior chest muscles. Due to poor flexor control, chronically ill children often are delayed in their ability to bring their hands to midline and to reach.

Encouraging midline skills in the small infant can be facilitated by placing the child in supine in the bed, on the floor, or the therapist's lap. The child's shoulder girdle, head, and neck should be brought into good alignment first. The infant's hands can be placed together and clasping of the hands can be encouraged. Placing a rattle in the midline for the child to reach for and hold also provides an opportunity to practice this skill. Toys with small rims or handles are easier for the infant to hold onto. Reaching can be encouraged through the use of a playgym or other mechanism for suspending toys. It is often helpful to place the child in a slightly reclined position rather than flat on the floor because gravity can assist in maintaining good shoulder position.

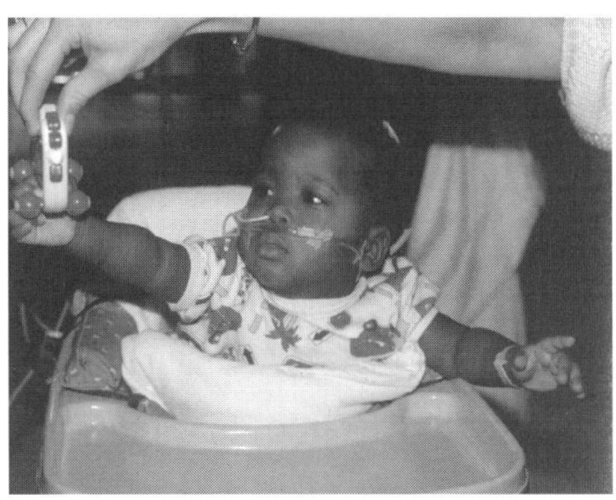

Side-lying is a good position in which to work on midline and reaching skills for infants and older children. Gravity assists in this position to keep the arms in midline and the chest muscles do not have to work against gravity. Side-lying is especially good for older children with neuromotor problems who are more difficult to position well in supine. Children with respiratory problems also tend to tolerate a side-lying position well. Toys should be presented as described above. Good side-lying positioning may require some of the adaptations described earlier.

Development of Weight-Bearing and Upright Postures

A large part of therapy is spent teaching children to sit, maintain quadruped, kneel, half-kneel, and stand. These positions require a significant amount of weight-bearing through the shoulder girdle and hips. Typically, children in the PICU have had limited exposure to such positions. They may be resistant to weight-bearing because of lack of experience. Weight-bearing, however, is crucial for promoting bone growth and maintaining bone integrity. There are many ways to promote weight-bearing through the extremities and in upright postures. A few suggestions will be offered in the following discussion. These suggestions are appropriate when children in the PICU are relatively stable. However, very few children in the acute phase of their illness can tolerate working on the more advanced skills beyond sitting, such as quadruped, kneeling, high kneeling, and standing.

Weight-bearing

Prone and sitting are good positions to facilitate **weight-bearing** through the shoulder girdle. *In prone*, the child can be placed over a bolster or wedge with her elbows or hands on the surface. Her shoulder girdle should be aligned directly above her elbows. The bolster or wedge provides support to the upper trunk. *In sitting*, the child can be encouraged to bear weight on her hands for support; or a small table can be placed in front of the child and she may be encouraged to bear weight through her elbows.

Positions that are useful for encouraging weight-bearing by the lower extremities include side-lying, sitting, and standing. To facilitate weight-bearing over the lower extremities while *in side-lying*, the child's upper leg should be flexed and externally rotated. The foot should be placed flat on the ground anterior to the child's body. The knees should be aligned directly above the ankles.

Lower extremity weight-bearing can be encouraged *in sitting* by placing the child on the interventionist's lap. The child's feet are placed flat on the ground with the hips, knees, and ankles flexed. Again the knee should be flexed directly over the ankle.

It is obvious that the *standing position* encourages lower extremity weight-bearing. If the child can stand by leaning against a support such as a small table, then this should be encouraged. However, many chronically ill children below age two years will not have achieved this level of motor control. Other options that encourage standing include prone or supine standers. The standers allow a child to stand supported in good postural alignment, while the therapist encourages the child to work on reaching for objects. The prone stander provides the support from the front while the supine stander provides the support from the back. If the child has poor head control, the supine stander may be a better option because the stander can be tilted backward in space allowing gravity to assist in keeping the head up. **No one should place a child in a stander without consultation from a physical therapist**.

The physical therapist should also be responsible for adjusting the stander to the appropriate size for the child.

Sitting

Sitting balance can be worked on in several ways. The normal progression of sitting is for the child to gain control in:

1) The anterior-posterior directions
2) The lateral direction
3) Into rotational patterns

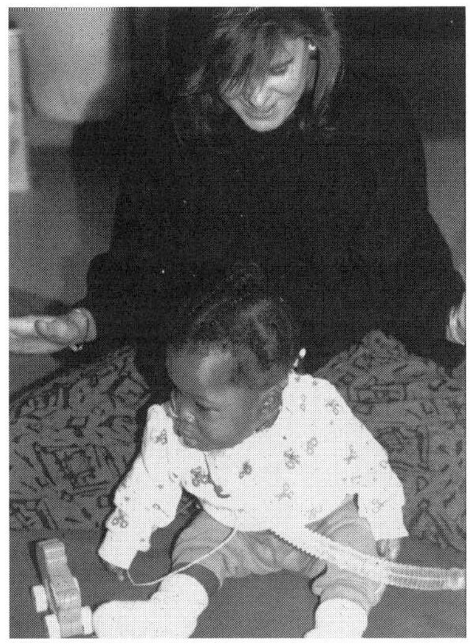

A good way to work on sitting is to place the child in a sitting posture on a floormat between the therapist's legs with the child's back to the therapist. The child should be given as much support as he needs for sitting. The child will first gain control in the **anterior-posterior directions**. The therapist works to establish control by facilitating movement in this direction. This can be done by placing a toy in front of the child, slightly out of his reach. The child then has to lean forward to get the toy and bring himself back to upright. As the child gains control of movement in this direction, he can be encouraged to move in the **lateral direction**. This can be facilitated by the use of a toy placed at the side of the child and slightly out of reach.

Once the child has improved in her ability to control her movements in the lateral direction, she can be encouraged to use **rotation** in her movements. The child should be encouraged to turn her trunk to obtain a toy. Rotation is important to enable the child to move in and out of sitting into other positions.

There are many choices when working on **sitting.** It is usually best to start working on the floor, as discussed above, as this allows the child the greatest base of support. However, as the child improves, sitting may be practiced on a variety of surfaces, such as *benches, bolsters, and balls.* **Benches** allow the child to work on sitting with a smaller base of support. The child may straddle the bench with the legs abducted, providing a relatively wide base of support, or he may be seated with both his feet on the same side of the bench. The child may first work on sitting on the bench using his hands for support. His hands may be placed on the bench or in front of him on another surface. An example of this would be to have the child seated on the bench in front of a mirror with his shoulders flexed at 90 degrees and elbows extended with his hands on the mirror for support. As the child improves and is able to sit independently on the bench, the therapist may challenge his balance by providing reaching activities in all planes of movement.

Bolsters allow the child to work on sitting balance with a moving surface. The child can be placed straddling the bolster or placed sitting with both feet on the same side. The amount of movement can be controlled by the therapist or by the child. Work on balance can occur in predictable and unpredictable situations addressing anticipatory and feedback responses as described previously.

Balls allow the child to practice sitting in very challenging positions. **The use of a ball for sitting should only be done under the close supervision of a physical**

therapist. The child can be placed in sitting on the ball with her feet supported on the floor, or the child can be held on the ball by the therapist without the feet supported. When the child is on the ball with the feet supported, she is able to use her legs to help her balance. This allows her to work on sitting balance and weight shifting in her pelvis and feet in all directions. The therapist provides the degree of support necessary for the child's abilities. When working on the ball without the feet supported, the therapist provides the support. However, the location on the child's body where the support is provided is dependent upon the abilities of the child. The child with poorer sitting balance will require more support in the trunk, while the child with better sitting balance may only require the therapist to hold her by her ankles.

Quadruped

Quadruped is another developmental position that the therapist may need to facilitate with chronically ill children. A good way to begin working on quadruped is over a bolster that allows the child's knees to make contact with the floor and allows his arms to extend with hands on the floor. The bolster supports the trunk. Once the child is placed in this position, the therapist can gently move the bolster back and forth so that the child gets the sensation of weight-bearing through his hips and shoulders. This allows a gradual adjustment to weight by the joints and helps to decrease resistance from the child. As the child learns to tolerate this and gains more control in his trunk, the therapist may switch to a smaller bolster, then just to hand support, and finally to independence. A small ball may also be used in teaching the child the quadruped position, but because the ball moves in many planes, it may be necessary to provide more support to the child than is necessary with a bolster.

High Kneeling

High kneeling is a position children typically move through to get to standing. It refers to kneeling with the hips extended. The therapist can work on high kneeling next to a small bench so that the arms are supported. This position allows the child to be upright while maintaining weight through her hips. As the child improves in this position, the therapist can have the child practice next to a bolster or ball. A technique to work on high kneeling that most children enjoy is to have the child face you and try to push you over while maintaining her balance in position.

Half-Kneeling

Half-kneeling is the position children typically move into from high kneeling when making a transition to standing. It refers to a position with one knee down and one knee up. It is more challenging than high kneeling because most of the child's weight is over one extremity. This is an important position to work on in therapy because it is part of the sequence in rising to a standing position.

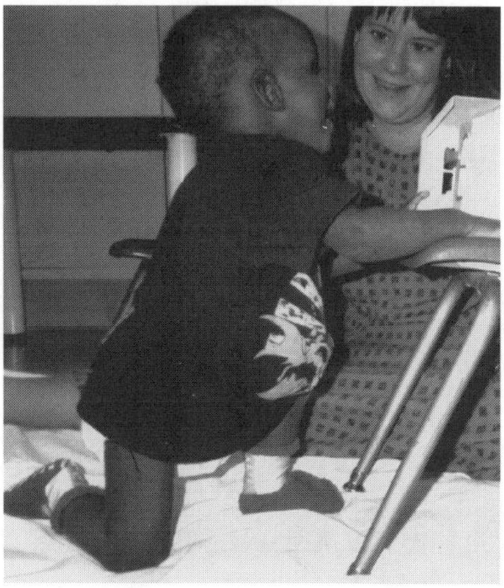

Standing

Standing is obviously an important skill. Independent standing is necessary for independent walking. The therapist can assist the child in standing by furniture or by supporting him as needed away from furniture. As the child learns to stand alone, the therapist can provide activities focusing on standing balance. Work on standing must be planned in conjunction with the child's readiness for this skill.

DEALING WITH OTHER COMMON NEUROMOTOR PROBLEMS

Autonomic Regulation

Chronically ill children often display difficulty maintaining good state organization. At times they may be irritable and hyperalert; at other times, somewhat unresponsive and lethargic. Vestibular input can help reduce these problems. Providing gentle movements in the vertical directions while holding the child securely may be a calming technique for the irritable child. For some infants, being snugly swaddled in a blanket has a calming effect and allows them to be more alert. For the lethargic child, brisk movement in a horizontal direction may make her more alert.

Tactile Defensiveness

Many chronically ill children display problems with tactile defensiveness. They appear to respond very negatively to touch. This may be due to the repetitive invasive medical procedures they have endured, or it may be a function of central nervous system irritability. Deep pressure in sensitive areas is often helpful in reducing tactile defensiveness. Exposure to a variety of textured materials may also serve to desensitize the child to contact with tactile stimuli.

Musculoskeletal Problems

Some children with chronic illness present musculoskeletal problems such as contractures of the joints. These may be due to congenital malformations or may result from restricted movement. Good positioning in the hospital and at home is the best way to avoid the development of joint limitation. The child should be provided a variety of positions throughout the day. A second approach to preventing or reducing contractures is through passive range of motion exercises. These can be carried out on a regular basis by the parents and the nursing staff with guidance from the physical therapist.

Use of Adaptive Equipment

The use of adaptive equipment has been prevalent throughout this discussion of physical therapy intervention. There are several important points to be kept in mind when using adaptive equipment:

1. No piece of adaptive equipment should be used without knowledge of its intended use and specific training in its use.
2. A child should never be left unattended in or on an adaptive piece of equipment.
3. Adaptive equipment should be modified only within the limits of the adjustable features included in the design constraints of the system. Parts of the adaptive equipment should not be removed or extra pieces added as this changes the original design and can present a risk for the child.
4. Equipment should be cleaned regularly.
5. Equipment should be stored in a safe place when not in use to prevent tampering.

A listing of suppliers of adaptive equipment is provided in Table 11.

Table 11
Pediatric Adaptive Equipment Suppliers

The Equipment Shop P.O. Box 33 Bedford, MA 10730 617-275-7681	Preston (for Tumbleform products) 60 Page Road Clifton, NJ 07012 800-631-7277
Flaghouse Special Populations 150 No. MacQuesten Pkwy. Mt. Vernon, NY 10550 800-221-5185	Rifton Route 213 Rifton, NY 12471 914-658-3141
Kaye Products, Inc. 535 Dimmocks Mill Rd. Hillsborough, NC 27278 919-732-6444	Therapy Skill Builders 3830 E. Bellevue P.O. Box 42050-C91 Tucson, Arizona 85733 602-323-7500

CARRY-OVER BY PARENTS AND MEDICAL/NURSING STAFF

For consistent gains to be achieved in motor development of chronically ill children, the motor intervention goals must be integrated into the care plan throughout the day. This requires parents and nursing staff to be familiar with the techniques being used to facilitate motor progress.

The most effective means for parents and nurses to learn motor intervention activities is for them to participate in the treatment sessions the PT provides for the child. It is helpful for the therapist to describe what to observe and how a particular activity addresses the child's neuromotor deficits. If it is not possible for the parents to be present during a session, videotaping is an option. In addition, therapeutic activities may be posted at the bedside as well as described in the medical chart. Instant camera pictures are helpful in conveying the intent of the activity more clearly. "Graffiti" sheets can be posted bedside. A graffiti page provides a means for parents, nurses, and other professionals to record their informal observation of the child in relation to suggested activities.

Overall, it is important for the physical therapist to continually reassess the child's strengths and needs relative to the child's medical condition. Changes in medical status have a profound effect on the neuromotor functioning of these children. In addition, communication should be maintained with other members of the interdisciplinary team so that motor goals are integrated with other developmental goals of the intervention program.

REFERENCES

Als, H. (1984). Manual for the naturalistic observation of newborn behavior (preterm and full-term). Unpublished manuscript. Child Development Unit Children's Hospital Medical Center, Boston, MA.

Als, H., Lawhon, G., Brown, E., Gibes, R., Duffy, F., McAnulty, G., & Blickman, J. (1986). Individualized behavioral and environmental care for the very low birth weight preterm infant at high risk for bronchopulmonary dysplasia: Neonatal intensive care unit and developmental outcome. *Pediatrics,* 6, 1123-1132.

Als, H., Lester, B., Tronick, E., and Brazelton,T. (1982). Towards a research instrument for the assessment of preterm infant's behavior (APIB). In H. Fitzgerald, B. Lester, & M. Yogman (Eds.) *Theory and Research in Behavioral Pediatrics,* (Vol. 1, pp.1-35). New York: Plenum Press.

Ballard, R. (1988). *Pediatric Care and the ICN Graduate.* New York: WB Saunders Co.

Bayley, N. (1969). *The Bayley Scales of Infant Development.* San Antonio,TX: Psychological Corp.

Bly, L. (1983). The components of normal movement during the first year of life and abnormal motor development. Birmingham, AL: Pittenger and Associates.

Brazelton, T.B. (1984). *Neonatal Behavioral Assessment Scale* (2nd ed.) Philadelphia: Lippincott.

Bzoch, K. & League, R. (1991). *Receptive and Expressive Emergent Language Scale.* Austin, TX: PRO-ED Inc.

Chandler, L., Andrews, M., & Swanson, M. (1980). *Movement Assessment of Infants. A Manual.* Rolling Bay, WA: Movement Assessment of Infants.

Cole, J. (1989). A nurture center for chronically ill infants. *American Journal of Nursing,* 89(8) 1062A, 1062E, 1062H.

Davis, B. & Steel, S. (1991). Case management for young children with special health care needs. *Pediatric Nursing,* 17(1), 15-19.

Dubowitz, L. & Dubowitz, V. (1981). The neurological assessment of the preterm and full-term newborn infant, *Clinics in Developmental Medicine,* No.79, Philadelphia: Lippincott.

Fewell, R. (1991). Trends in the assessment of infants and toddlers with disabilities. *Exceptional Children,* 58(2), pp. 166-173.

Folio, M. & Fewell, R. (1983). *Peabody Developmental Motor Scales and Activity Cards.* Allen, TX: Teaching Resources.

Furuno, S., Inatsuka, T., O'Reilly, K., Hosaka, C., Zeisloft, B. & Allman,T. (1984). *HELP Checklist* (Hawaii Early Learning Profile). Palo Alto, CA: VORT Corp.

Griffiths, R. (1976). *The Abilities of Babies.* High Wycombe, England: The Test Agency LTD.

Hedrick, D., Prather, E., & Tobin, A. (1984). *Sequenced Inventory of Communicative Development - Revised.* Seattle: University of Washington.

Johnson-Martin, N., Jens, K., and Attermeier, S. (1986). *The Carolina Curriculum for Handicapped Infants and Infants At Risk.* Baltimore: P.H. Brookes.

Kaufman, A. & Kaufman, N. (1983) *Kaufman Assessment Battery for Children.* Circle Pine, MN: American Guidance Service.

Knobloch, H., Stevens, F., & Malone, A. (1980). *Manual of Developmental Diagnosis for the Administration and Interpretation of the Revised Gesell and Amatruda Developmental and Neurological Examination.* Hagerstown, MD: Harper and Son.

McCarthy, D. (1972). *McCarthy Scales of Childrens' Abilities.* San Antonio, TX: Psych. Corp.

Montgomery, P.C., & Connally, B.H. (1991). *Motor Control and Physical Therapy* (1st ed.). Hixon, TN: Chattanooga Group Inc.

Nickel, R., Penken, C., & Gallenstein, J. (1989). The infant motor screen. *Developmental Medicine and Child Neurology.* 31, pp. 35-42.

Pearson, P. (1975). *A Manual of the Milani-Comparetti Testing Prodecure.* Omaha: University of Nebraska Medical Center.

Perrin, E. & Gerrity, S. (1984). Development of children with a chronic illness. *Pediatric Clinics of North America,* 31(1), pp. 19-31.

Ramsay, M. and Fitzhardinge, P. (1977). A comparative study of two developmental scales: The Bayley and the Griffiths. *Early Human Development,* 1(2), pp. 151-157.

Reynell, J. (1977). *Reynell Developmental Language Scales.* Slough, Buckinghamshire. N.F.E.R.

Reynell, J. (1979). *The Reynell-Zinkin Scales: Developmental scales for young visually handicapped children.* Windsor, England: NFER Publishing.

Richardson, J. & Robinson, S. (1989). Neonatal intensive care and pediatric rehabilitation: A joint program for care of chronically ill infants. *Journal of Perinatology,* 9(1), pp.52-55.

Shelton, T., Jeppson, E., & Johnson, B. (1987). *Family Centered Care for Children with Special Health Care Needs.* Washington, DC: Association for the Care of Children's Health.

Simeonsson, R., Huntington, G., Short, R., & Ware, W. (1982). The Carolina Record of Infant Behavior: Characteristics of handicapped infants and children. *Topics in Early Childhood Special Education.* 2, pp.43-55.

Sparrow, S., Ballo, D., & Cicchetti, D. (1984). *The Vineland Adaptive Behavior Scales.* Circle Pines, MN: American Guidance Service.

Stillman, R. (1978). *The Callier-Azusa Scale.* Dallas: University of Texas.

Stutsman, R. (1931). *Merrill Palmer Scale of Mental Tests.* Chicago: C.H. Stoelting, Co.

Tecklin, J.S. (Ed.). (1989). *Pediatric Physical Therapy.* Philadelphia, PA: J.B. Lippincott Co.

Thorndike, R., Hagen, E., & Sattler, J. (1986). *Stanford Binet Intelligence Scale* (4th ed). Chicago: Riverside.

Uzgiris, I. & Hunt, J. (1975). *Assessment in Infancy: Ordinal Scales of Psychological Development.* Urbana: University of Illinois Press.

Vessey, J., Risom, L. & Farley, J. (1991). Iatrogenic developmental effects of pediatric intensive care. *Pediatric Nursing,* 17(3), pp. 12-15.

Wolfer, J., Gayhard, L., Goldberger, J., & Laidley, L. (1989). *Helping Children and Families Cope with Hospitalization: An Integration of Theory and Clinical Practice.* Washington, DC: Association for the Care of Children's Health.

Chapter 5

The Impact of Chronic Illness on Communication Development and Feeding

Sharon Willig, M.A., CCC-SLP

The role of a speech-language pathologist (SLP) on an inpatient developmental team focuses frequently on providing input related to oral-motor functioning and feeding. The SLP meets with the family of the infant and their medical/nursing caregivers to determine their priorities in facilitating the infant's management during that admission. Although feeding problems are most frequently the reason for SLP referrals, social communication needs are simultaneously addressed and made part of the oral-motor/feeding program.

The information covered in this chapter is designed to provide:

1) An overview of factors that place an infant at risk for a communication disorder
2) A framework for assessment
3) Rationales for providing intervention

Oral-motor and feeding issues will be targeted areas.

IDENTIFYING COMMUNICATION DISORDERS AND FEEDING PROBLEMS

Young children with chronic illness frequently demonstrate factors that put them at risk for:

- Hearing loss
- Language delay
- Oral-motor problems
- Speech disorders
- Social communication deficits

The lifesaving medications and technologies used during early infancy may contribute to adverse conditions affecting later communication skill development and feeding.

HEARING PROBLEMS

To initiate the necessary medical and educational intervention for developing optimal communication and social skills, the early detection of hearing impairment in children is essential. Familiarity with risk factors will enable hospital and early intervention staff to assist in early identification of hearing problems. The criteria for neonates (birth to 28 days) and infants (29 days to two years) that places them at risk for sensorineural hearing impairment are listed in Table 12.

Table 12
Risk Criteria for Neonates and Infants At Risk for Sensorineural Hearing Impairment
(Joint Committee on Infant Hearing, 1991)

Neonates (birth - 28 days)	Infants (29 days - 2 years)
• Family history of congenital or delayed onset childhood sensorineural hearing impairment	• Parent/caregiver concern regarding hearing, speech, language, and/or developmental delay
• Congenital infection known or suspected to be associated with sensorineural hearing impairment, such as toxoplasmosis, syphillis, rubella, cytomegalovirus and herpes	• Bacterial meningitis
• Craniofacial anomalies including morphologic abnormalities of the pinna and ear canal, absent philtrum, low hairline, etc.	• Neonatal risk factors listed in the adjacent column
• Birthweight less than 1500 grams (3.3 pounds)	• Head trauma
• Hyperbilirubinemia at a level exceeding indication for exchange transfusion	• Syndromes known to include sensorineural hearing loss (e.g., Waardenburg or Ushers Syndrome)
• Ototoxic medications including gentamicin, tobramycin, kanamycin, streptomycin (used for more than five days)	• Ototoxic medications as listed in the adjacent column
• Bacterial meningitis	• Children with neurodegenerative disorders such as neurofibromatosis, Werdnig-Hoffman disease, Tay-Sachs disease, infantile Gaucher's disease, Nieman-Pick disease
• Severe depression at birth, which may include infants with Apgar score of 0-3 at 5 minutes or those who fail to initiate spontaneous respiration by 10 minutes or those with hypotonia persisting to 2 hours of age	• Childhood infectious diseases known to be associated with sensorineural hearing loss (e.g., mumps, measles)
• Prolonged mechanical ventilation for a duration equal to or greater than 10 days (e.g. persistent pulmonary hypertension)	
• Stigmata or other findings associated with a syndrome known to include sensorineural hearing loss	

Neonates who manifest one or more risk factors should be screened for hearing function by an audiologist prior to discharge from the newborn nursery but no later than three months of age. Older infants who exhibit one or more risk factors should be screened for hearing function within three months of the child's identification as at-risk. Procedures used by audiologists to assess hearing are described in Appendix A.

Hearing screening has often been limited to the infants who reside in the NICU, which accounts for only one-third of the children later identified as having hearing loss. The newest guidelines expand the risk criteria for screening in an effort to include more of the group that has historically been untested at the earliest stages. When hearing loss is present, other disabilities, such as mental retardation, learning disabilities, attention deficits, vestibular deficits, behavior disorders, and visual deficits may also be present (Goudreau et al., 1989; Karchmer, 1985).

Many tertiary care hospitals follow protocols for evaluating infants' hearing status prior to discharge. However, as infants may be transferred from one hospital to another, one cannot assume hearing was evaluated early on or reevaluated following the use of medications known to have ototoxic side effects. The interventionist has the responsibility to question the primary physician or the parent regarding hearing screening and to request that hearing be tested if no previous report is available.

An infant with identified hearing loss is eligible for early intervention services in accordance with IDEA Part H. Infants with seriously impaired hearing may be candidates for amplification and/or alternative/augmentative communication strategies, e.g., total communication.

LANGUAGE PROBLEMS

Normal language development is dependent upon an intact peripheral nervous system, an intact central nervous system, favorable environmental factors, normal intelligence, a good health status, and emotional stability. As problems in one or more of the aforementioned areas put a child at risk for a language delay, most children with chronic illness are at risk.

Assessment of infant communication skills focuses primarily on each child's interactions with her environment. Behavioral observations of the infant's responses to stimulation, her strategies to alert caregivers of a need, the infant's pleasure/displeasure signals, her adaptation to new situations, and her play skills provide the clinician with information to determine communication styles and developmental levels. The clinician assesses the ways in which the infant comprehends and uses language at the pre-verbal and verbal stages. Assessment measures frequently used by pediatric speech-language pathologists are listed in Appendix A.

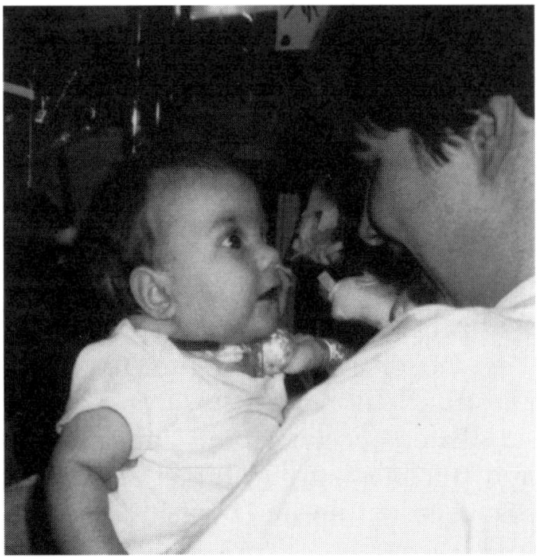

Once a developmental assessment is completed, language goals can be integrated into the overall intervention plan. Recommended goals for the chronically ill infants will often target the following areas:

- Enhancing auditory-visual interaction
- Providing opportunities for communication
- Facilitating responses from infants

Alternative/augmentative communication aids and/or toys to assist in program implementation may be made available to the parents and the medical/nursing staff by the interventionist. It is preferable if communication goals can be integrated into caregiving activities, such as feeding or changing diapers. Suggestions to modify the infant's environment to make it more conducive to social interaction may be helpful. These might include the following:

- Turning off the television
- Closing the room door to reduce the noise from the hallway
- Reducing bright light from the windows and ceiling lights
- Scheduling "social play times" when no procedures are anticipated

ORAL-MOTOR/FEEDING PROBLEMS

Feeding difficulties are common in infants and young children with chronic respiratory problems, congenital cardiac defects, central nervous system dysfunction or other chronic illnesses.

The typical oral/motor/feeding problems these children exhibit include:

- Weak suck
- Inefficient suck-swallow patterns
- Poor coordination of suck-swallow with breathing
- Emesis
- Inactive cheek/lip musculature
- Tongue retraction
- Jaw thrusting

Medical procedures themselves may complicate the establishment of normal feeding. Prolonged endotracheal intubation and the use of orogastric or nasogastric tubes for gavage feeding further disorganize the oral-feeding mechanism. During hospitalization, the pleasant feelings usually associated with feeding are often disrupted as are the normal bonding and communicative behaviors for both the infants and the caregivers.

A full discussion of assessment and intervention strategies for feeding problems follows later in this chapter.

SPEECH PROBLEMS

Speech production is essentially a voluntary motor act dependent upon the normal functioning and coordination of the following speech mechanisms:

- Respiration
- Phonation
- Resonation
- Articulation
- The oral-peripheral structures

Any alteration to this fine-tuned system can interfere with speech production. The speech system frequently becomes disturbed in the technology-dependent, chronically ill population.

Later, speech production of a chronically ill child is often affected by intubation and tracheostomy (a direct airhole into the trachea) that have provided the airway management needed by a child with respiratory difficulties. When endotracheal intubation and mechanical ventilation are necessary, the infant is at risk for complications, such as vocal fold paralysis. Bilateral vocal fold paralysis in the open position—abductor paralysis—can interfere with the infant's ability to synchronize respiration with feeding, resulting in aspiration. Vocal folds in the closed position—adductor paralysis—interferes with respiration.

Voice quality is determined by the adequacy of the vocal fold closure, the coordination of vocal fold closure with exhalation, and the amount of muscle tone present in the laryngeal area (Alexander, 1983). Children who are dependent upon cannulation (airway management by tube) during and beyond the prelingual period (more than six months) may not achieve normal anatomic and physiologic development of the speech mechanism. When decannulated, alterations of the vocal tract anatomy and physiology may result in poor vocal fold functioning and abnormal muscle tone in the laryngeal area (Alexander, 1983; Kamen and Watson, 1991). The voice quality may be characterized by a tense, hoarse, breathy or rattling sound. Maladaptive oral-motor compensations during cannulation can result in altered articulatory movements for speech following decannulation.

Speech production can be enhanced or augmented by use of computer technology, sign language, speech valves, object/picture boards, and electro-larynxs for infants who require tracheostomies for prolonged periods of time.

SOCIAL COMMUNICATION PROBLEMS

Social communication may be affected by a child's emotional and developmental well-being. During hospitalization, the child's emotional functioning may be affected by the following environmental threats:

1) Multiple caregivers
2) Lack of diurnal rhythm (lack of mealtime and bedtime ritual behaviors)
3) Immobility/confinement
4) Medical equipment
5) Painful procedures
6) Mechanical feeding procedures
7) Noncontingent interactions
8) Inappropriate stimulation

(Goldberger and Wolfer, 1991)

Any one of these "threats" can have a negative impact on the ecological balance involved in the child's behavioral homeostasis, attachment, and separation.

Infants experiencing environmental stress exhibit problems in feeding, sleep, mood, self-consoling, arousal, and transitions. Infants may show maladaptive behaviors, such as:

- Not visually engaging
- Not smiling
- Not vocalizing reciprocally
- Not reaching out in anticipation when picked up
- Lack of cuddling when held
- Refusal behaviors (e.g. feeding refusals)

(Chatoor, 1991)

FEEDING PROBLEMS IN INFANTS

Maintaining adequate nourishment is the second of the two major physical needs of medically fragile children. Promoting normal respiration is the primary need. In this section, the normal feeding experiences for infants will be reviewed. Secondly, assessment and intervention strategies with chronically ill children will be discussed.

Impact of the NICU/PICU Environment on Feeding

The normal infant associates feeding and sucking with comfortable, pleasurable experiences. When held closely, the child makes eye contact with the caregiver's face, feels contentment, and develops positive socially communicative responses, such as cooing, smiling, and looking. Body adjustments in response to her caregiver and the satisfaction of feeling full teach the young child that feeding is a positive experience. Such experiences foster healthy relationships among the infant, the caregiver, and the environment.

In the normal infant, sucking patterns are efficiently organized with suck, swallow and respiration occurring in a synchronized sequence. The infant is flexible in adjusting the suck to the demands of the situation.

Many factors associated with intensive medical care and treatment of serious illness can delay and interfere with the development of normal feeding patterns.

Feeding small, preterm infants and some medically fragile older infants requires specialized techniques somewhat different than breast- or bottle-feeding a healthy, term infant. The infants with special needs have a number of problems that complicate feeding. Frequently, their gastrointestinal tracts are immature and unable to accept and digest adequate quantities of food. *Intravenous feeding (TPN or total parenteral nutrition)* of specially prepared solutions helps provide satisfactory amounts of most nutrients. When medications cannot be accepted by the digestive tract, the infant may also be provided TPN ingestion through insertion of a broviac catheter into a major vein. As the infant's gastrointestinal tract matures and satisfactory weight gain occurs, *enteral feedings* (feedings given into the gastrointestinal tract either by mouth and/or by tube) gradually replace parenteral feedings (intravenous feedings). The tube feedings may be nasogastric, orogastric, transpyloric, jejunal or by gastrostomy. Hypersensitivity to touch to the face may result from:

- Prolonged exposure to the gavage feeding tubes
- Tape on the face to hold tubing
- Endotracheal tubes
- Tracheostomies and suctioning
- Unpleasant-tasting medications

The infant who is exposed to pain paired frequently with noxious oral stimuli begins to respond negatively to any oral stimuli.

Sensory overstimulation (auditory, visual, and tactile) may interfere with the infant's ability to organize movements and coordination for efficient feeding. Studies of the NICU have shown it to be an overstimulating environment (Bess et al, 1979). Measures of ambient noise in the NICU have found that levels may be high enough to damage the immature cochlea. In addition to disrupting feeding, these noise levels may alter sleep states, producing increased active sleep rather than deep sleep. Apnea occurs more frequently during active sleep and can lead to hypoxemia.

In addition to high levels of stimulation, the hospitalized infant must follow a schedule imposed by adults regardless of the infant's state of arousal and readiness for interaction, feeding or medical procedures. The sensory overstimulation combined with the daily multiple changes in caregivers creates inconsistencies which make learning difficult. The individual differences among caregivers tends to disorganize sensory experiences for this young population.

Immaturity of the central nervous system in premature and chronically ill children may also contribute to feeding problems. These youngsters lack energy for feeding and are often fatigued before they can consume adequate amounts of formula or solids. Their low energy level and their respiratory illnesses interfere with the coordination needed for sucking, swallowing, and breathing.

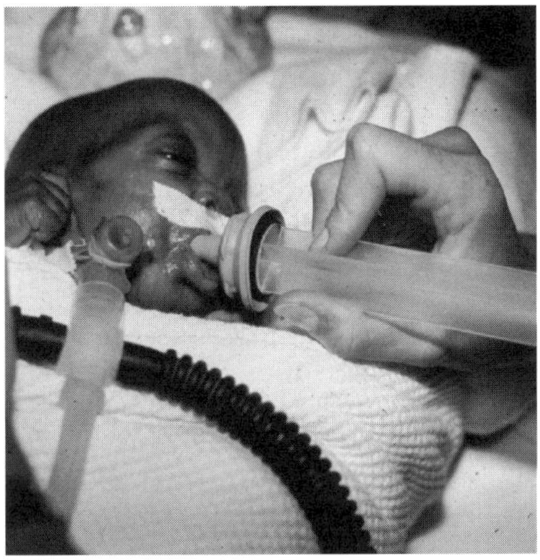

The introduction to oral feeding for hospitalized infants may begin when the infant's medical state is stabilized and weight gain has been adequately maintained by tube feeding. A conducive infant state or level of arousal must be present, and the infant's ability to tolerate nippling should be established (VandenBerg, 1990). The suck-swallow, breathing coordination does not usually mature until at least 34+ weeks gestational age. Although some infants younger than 34 weeks gestational age demonstrate the ability to feed, they are at a higher risk for aspiration.

The following may contribute to common feeding problems of premature or chronically ill infants:

- Abnormal muscle tone
- Lack of proximal stability of the neck, shoulders, and trunk
- Exaggerated extensor patterns of movement
- Irritability
- Weak oral reflexes
- Limited tongue mobility
- An inadequate lip seal
- Poor cheek stability
- Oral hypersensitivity due to enteral tube feedings
- A disorganized suck-swallow-breathe pattern
- Prolonged use of endotracheal tubes, resulting in hyperextension and deviations of vocal quality.

(Morris and Klein, 1987)

Although nonnutritive sucking is encouraged in prematures before oral feeding is introduced, some infants have a poor ability to shift from nonnutritive to nutritive sucking (VandenBerg, 1990). Earlier studies by Braun and Palmer (1982) and Harris (1986) found that nutritive sucking differs from nonnutritive in that, in mature infants, nutritive sucking has bursts of longer duration than nonnutritive patterns and thus appears slower. Palmer (1989) concluded that infants who cannot shift and change their rate of sucking may have a neurologically-based problem.

Oral-Motor/Feeding Assessments

When initiating an oral-motor evaluation and/or a feeding assessment, the clinician should review the infant's medical chart, regarding:

- Birth history
- Health history
- Developmental history
- Feeding history

Gestational age, birth weight, perinatal complications, medical diagnosis, and hospitalization history should be considered by the clinician in evaluating needs. The type and frequency of medications the child receives should be noted, along with their manner of ingestion, e.g. orally, intravenously, etc. Many medications have side effects that may influence appetite, level of irritability, gastrointestinal tract functioning, muscle tone and/or alertness. If a child has been intubated, the type of intubation and the length of time intubated may also affect current functioning.

It is important to document the presenting feeding problem, the child's feeding schedule, how long the presenting feeding problem has been identified, the methods previously used to alleviate the problem, and the findings of other specialists who have also been consulted regarding the same problem. Nursing notes and consult sheets usually provide this information. The formula, the kinds of nipples used, length of time required for feeding, and any adjustments or changes the various caregivers have been implementing need to be investigated.

An oral-motor reflex assessment may precede a feeding observation. The inappropriate absence or presence of some reflexes can have a negative impact on feeding proficiency. The infant's communication skill levels should also be documented. Recommendations and follow-up should occur as part of an interdisciplinary effort to prioritize the infant's needs.

The *oral reflex exam* assesses age-expected (corrected for prematurity) reflexes and may include:

- Rooting
- Suckling
- Sucking
- Mouth opening
- Cardinal points
- The bite reflex
- The gag

(Blager, 1982)

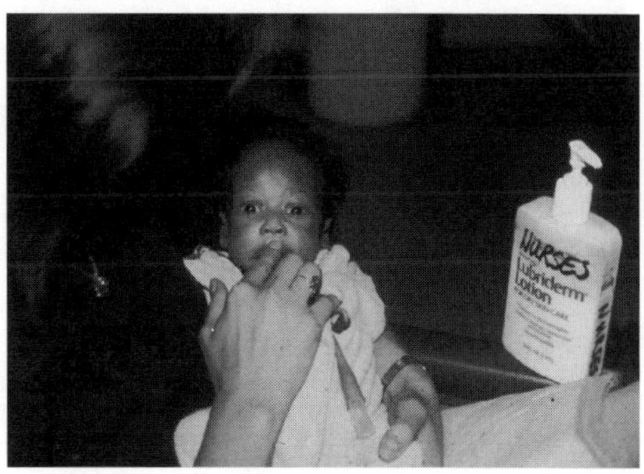

The feeding assessment should include *behavioral observations* regarding:

- The infant's state
- Caregiver's responses
- The infant's tolerance for being handled
- The infant's position during feeding

This kind of observation can provide the clinician with information regarding sensorimotor and communication problems related to feeding.

During oral feeding, the SLP checks symmetry of the oral musculature and notes the infant's movements and control of the lips, cheeks, jaw, and tongue. Any structural anomalies of the oral-peripheral mechanism are noted. Oral-motor muscle tone and strength and rhythm of the suck is assessed by having the infant suck on the clinician's finger (digital stimulation). The types of food offered, their textures and temperatures are also documented. As hospital-based caregiving usually involves the necessity for multiple feeders, a hands-on evaluation by the feeding specialist is not always recommended unless the clinician can be available for several consecutive feeding sessions. Infants demonstrate many stress behaviors during feeding that investigators have found relate to differences in styles of caregiver handling. Changes in autonomic, motor, and state behaviors have been described in disorganized infant feeders. Providing consistent caregivers fosters familiarity and predictability and is valuable when evaluating and regulating feeding behaviors. When time is not available for an ongoing assessment over several consecutive feeding sessions, a clinician can frequently determine feeding strengths and needs through interviewing and observing the primary caregivers prior to and during a feeding situation.

Based on Imhoff and Wigginton (1991), the information the SLP hopes to obtain through the feeding assessment includes the following:

- The child's level of alertness
- Postural tone
- Head and trunk control
- Response to touch on the body, face, and mouth
- Oral reflexes
- Suck-swallow-breathe coordination
- The strength, duration and rhythm of the suck
- The presence or absence of drooling
- Lip, tongue, and jaw control related to cup-drinking, spoon-feeding, biting, and chewing.

For children who demonstrate self-feeding skills, clinical observation should also include:

- Hand-to-mouth coordination
- Utensils used
- Oral-motor function
- Willingness to try new foods
- Efficiency
- Oral play and exploration

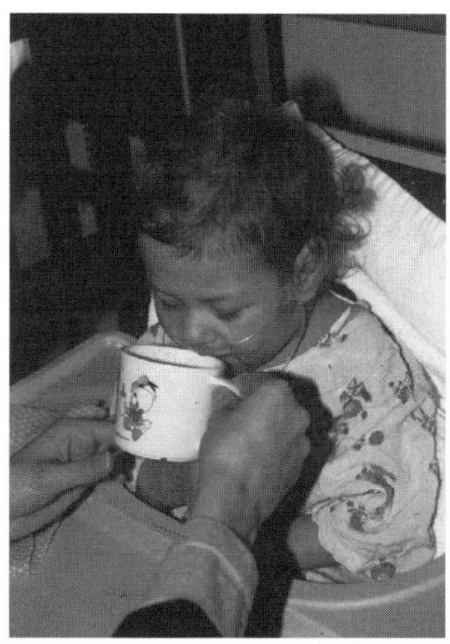

When the infant's clinical evaluation and physical history suggest possible aspiration, a pediatric oral-pharyngeal motility (OPM - video- swallow) study should be performed by a pediatric radiologist and an SLP. This assessment will analyze the interaction of feeding, swallowing, and respiration. It will determine if oral feeding is safe for the infant.

A "blue dye" study may be performed to assess airway safety in children who have a tracheostomy tube. This technique involves injecting a blue dye in food or liquid and having the child swallow it. The presence of blue secretions in the tracheostomy or seen by suctioning the child after the feeding indicates aspiration has occurred.

Tube Feeding

When an alternative or adjunctive method to oral feeding is needed, the feeding options include the following:

- **Parenteral** - feeding through a vein
- **Enteral** - feeding through the gastrointestinal route by tube

Parenteral nutrition is used with prematures or sick infants who are ill-equipped to maintain constant blood sugar levels during times of fasting and/or have renal problems which interfere with the maintenance of normal body electrolytes. Since a fairly constant supply of fluid, glucose, and electrolytes is necessary for survival, parenteral nutrition by vein is used with this population. When given through a small vein, it is called peripheral hyperalimentation. When a large catheter is inserted through a large vein, it is called central hyperalimentation. Although parenteral nutrition is essential in infants unable to tolerate feeding, it has serious side effects. The side effects can include the following:

- IV infiltrations and tissue damage similar to burns
- Sepsis
- Blockage of the major vessels from a clot formation

Enteral nutrition by tube is provided when there is some physical or anatomical reason why a child cannot get enough calories by mouth to provide adequate nutrition. Children may be prescribed enteral tube feeding in conjunction with one or more of the following problems:

- Prematurity
- Severe diarrhea
- Inability to suck
- Neurological impairments
- Cardiac problems
- Chronic pulmonary disease

Infants who breathe at rates greater than 60 to 80 times per minute will not feed well. Immature or ill infants often demonstrate poor coordination of sucking with breathing which causes them to become apneic and cyanotic during feeding. Severe birth asphyxia or prolonged intubation also contribute to problems tolerating oral feeding.

The various types of tube feeding routes used include the following:

- Orogastric - a tube through the mouth into the stomach
- Nasogastric - a tube through the nose into the stomach
- Transpyloric - a tube crossing the pyloric exit of the stomach (may be oral or nasal)
- Jejunal - a tube ending in the jejunum (may be oral or nasal)
- Gastrostomy - a tube through the abdominal wall directly into the stomach.

The decision as to which tube to use is based on several factors, including the projected length of use and physiologic concerns. For infants who are likely to be on tube feeding for three or more months, a surgically implanted tube (e.g. gastrostomy) may be preferable in order to facilitate a more natural nasal-oral-pharyngeal environment for acquisition of oral feeding and/or oral stimulation experiences. Some complications associated with tube feeding include dislodgement, discomfort associated with insertion or removal, and tube blockage. Feeding therapists cite long-term use of orogastric tubes as major contributors to gagging, desensitization of the mouth, incomplete lip closure, and ineffective oral suck. Prolonged use of nasogastric tubes contributes to nasal obstruction and desensitization of the nasal-velar-pharyngeal areas. Although the gastrostomy involves an invasive surgical procedure for children who will require long-term enteral nutrition by tube, it does allow the child to experience more pleasurable oral experiences within a natural oral environment.

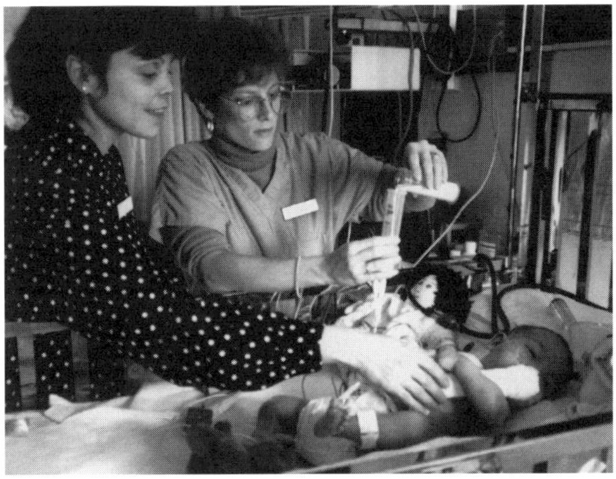

INTERDISCIPLINARY FEEDING INTERVENTION

The type of oral-motor and/or feeding treatment and timing of treatment for children with feeding problems involves the management, coordination, and cooperation of the family and the other members of the medical/habilitative care team. The composition of the team changes frequently, depending on the status and needs of the child and the family. Individuals in a hospital setting who might be involved in developing a feeding plan include:

- The family, who are ultimately responsible for the management and provision of overall caregiving
- The primary physician, who is responsible for the physical and medical well-being of the child
- The nutritionist, who supervises the dietary/nutritional aspects of the child's treatment
- The speech-language pathologist, who provides input regarding stimulation for oral-motor and communication development
- The lactation specialist, who facilitates mothers who wish to breast feed or use breast milk
- The occupational or physical therapist, who provides assistance for positioning and/or decreasing tactile defensiveness
- The nurse, who is responsible for the day-to-day medical monitoring and caregiving, including feeding
- The social worker, who works with families and medical personnel surrounding family needs and issues
- The infant development specialist, who provides stimulation to enhance cognitive development
- The pediatric psychologist who may assist in understanding behavioral aspects of the feeding problem

With so many individuals potentially involved, it is important for team members to meet routinely at least once a week, determine the infant's and family's needs and priorities, and identify the primary caregiver handlers. Ideally, the therapists serve as consultants to the family/medical care team and train them to employ techniques that will enhance the infant's learning and facilitate development of oral-motor function and feeding. Sick infants respond poorly to frequent changes in caregiver handling. The more consistent the handling in an habilitation program, perhaps, the speedier the response to therapeutic input.

MAJOR ELEMENTS OF A TREATMENT PLAN

In planning an oral-motor stimulation and/or feeding treatment program, each of the following areas must be considered:

- Caregiver consistency
- Environment
- Positioning
- Length/frequency/timing of feeds
- Infant states
- Feeding equipment
- Timing of therapeutic input

CAREGIVER CONSISTENCY

Most hospitals today cannot guarantee consistent nurse staffing patterns to facilitate feeding development in each child. Creative approaches to enhance consistency are needed. Parents need encouragement to come for regularly scheduled feeding times each day and to provide, with therapeutic guidance, the appropriate oral-motor experiences for their children. This may mean coming to the hospital for one or more feedings a day. To meet the needs of chronically ill children whose parents are not able to visit routinely, some hospitals are training volunteer grandparents, nursing students or other long-term trainees who are available on a daily basis for at least one feeding.

It is important for feeding teams to designate a minimum number of primary infant "handlers." When appropriate, a consultative therapeutic model may be established. The therapist instructs the handlers (parents, nurses, volunteers, etc.) in techniques for normalizing feeding. Limiting the number of handlers strengthens the infant's ability to adapt to the style of his primary feeder. A consultative approach is used successfully for many children who demonstrate the need for environmental adaptations. However, for children with neuromotor dysfunction and respiratory problems, there may be no substitute for direct therapeutic intervention. The therapeutic priorities for each child must be established by the child's medical/habilitative team.

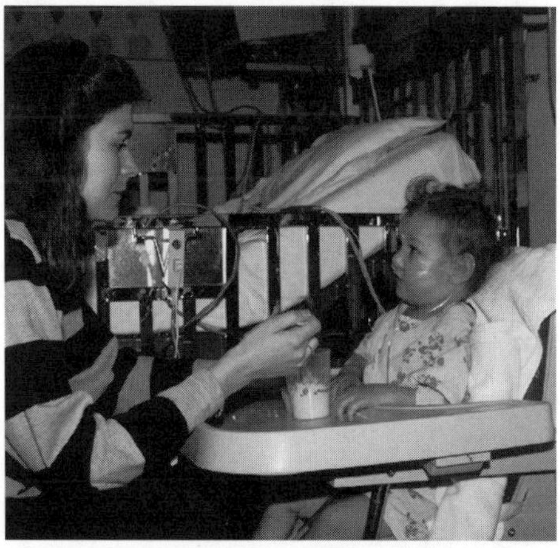

ENVIRONMENT

As discussed earlier in this chapter, the NICU and PICU are frequently overstimulating centers of activity. Bright lights, beeping monitors, invasive procedures, noisy radios/televisions, conversational speech, inconsistent comforting, and noxious stimuli interfere with an infant's ability to attend to and organize her world. Many infants "shut down" and fall asleep in an effort to escape.

In most instances, the SLP and the medical/habilitative team are jointly able to develop some positive adjustments to the feeding/pre-feeding environment, which include the following:

- Decreasing unnecessary auditory and visual stimulation by turning off the television, dimming the lights, and finding a quiet corner for rocking and holding the baby
- Avoiding stimulating procedures, such as chest PT or any potentially aversive handling within 30 minutes of feeding/oral-motor time
- Withdrawing the pacifier 20 minutes prior to feeding (unless the infant becomes irritable) to minimize sucking fatigue

Each hospital-based situation will present a variety of challenges. People working together can bring about environmental improvements.

POSITIONING

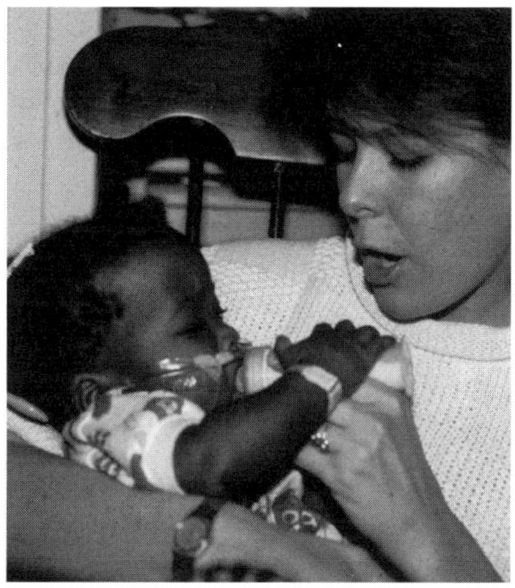

In most instances, holding a young infant is the preferred manner for all feedings. Whether the feeding is by mouth or tube, the element of warm human contact cannot be emphasized enough. It assists the infant in forming an attachment to the caregiver.

For a host of reasons, many infants with chronic illness demonstrate irritability and frequently manifest disorganized oral-motor movements. For their feeding times, firm swaddling is highly recommended. Bringing the child's arms to midline seems to calm sick infants and appears to help many infants focus their attention on the task at hand.

For infants three- to five-months of age and older without tracheostomies, a forward head tilt or chin tuck should be encouraged to facilitate their swallowing. This can be achieved by cuddling the baby with the head maintained in an upright position or by positioning the child in a chair so that the trunk and pelvis are in an alignment that maximizes normalization of muscle tone. Morris and Klein (1987) demonstrate a variety of positions that may facilitate oral-motor input and/or feeding. The occupational or physical therapist can aid the team in developing optimal and comfortable positions for the infant and the feeder.

LENGTH, FREQUENCY, AND TIME OF FEEDINGS:

A feeding goal is to have five scheduled feeding times during the day that would be comparable to three meals and two snacks. Enteral tube feedings for young infants are frequently regulated by a pump and take approximately one or more hours. If a pump is needed for an infant who can tolerate intake over shorter periods of time, the goal should be eventually to shorten feedings (oral and tube) to the time it would take a health baby to feed (20 minutes). This helps establish a meal routine and also allows the infant to experience levels of hunger and satiation. Additional nutrition needs can frequently be pumped at night.

When it is safe to feed orally, attempts at oral feeding should precede each tube feeding. Caution should be taken to avoid overly fatiguing the infant. Adequate opportunities to experience oral intake of feedings must be provided; yet the infant should be allowed to terminate feeding at any time. Many infants with respiratory problems and/or reflux have difficulty adhering to a strict feeding schedule. Some youngsters can only take small amounts of food at any one time. They require shorter, more frequent feeding opportunities.

Some infants who begin to tolerate oral feedings respond well to having their N/G tubes pulled for daytime "meals" and are supplemented by a reinserted tube only at night. This permits normalized oral-feeding experiences, even though their intake may be limited.

For infants who tolerate limited or no oral feedings, a pacifier, digital or breast stimulation may be accepted in and around the oral cavity during daytime tube feedings. This may help the child learn to associate pleasant oral sensations with the feeling of having a full stomach.

INFANT STATES

Successful oral feeding demands an alert, stable, hungry, and cooperative infant. Some chronically ill infants take up to one hour to become aroused, and some never completely wake up for their feeding times. The feeder needs to learn the individual infant's biorhythms and develop a schedule to facilitate optimal arousal.

A distressed, irritable infant will require time to calm down prior to oral-motor stimulation. Nonnutritive sucking on a pacifier, swaddling, cuddling, and rocking may help. Assisting the infant to get her hands to midline or to her mouth may permit self-comforting to occur.

FEEDING EQUIPMENT

For pre-feeding, oral-motor preparation, the feeder's hands are the most useful tools available. Many infants demonstrate tactile defensiveness learned from hospital procedures they have had to endure. One technique used to decrease tactile defensiveness is deep pressure massage. The application involves giving the infant a firm massage, starting with the feet and slowly working up the body to the face. Appropriate body alignment and tone normalization should be facilitated before using any oral stimulation. A skilled therapist can provide this intervention.

Formula-filled syringes or straws, fingers dipped in formula, wet washcloths, or pacifiers dipped in formula and touched to the infant's lips may be used to alert the infant of the upcoming feeding event. The infant's responses to stimulation should always be respected.

Different types of nipples are available to use with infants at various stages of development. Premature infants, infants with craniofacial anomalies and chronically ill infants frequently need commercially available nipples or adapted nipples to facilitate their feeds.

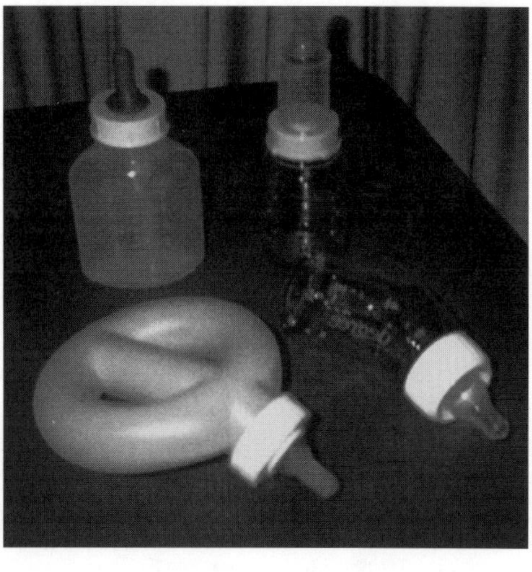

Parents of chronically ill infants who require frequent re-admissions to the hospital are a valuable resource for determining the appropriate nipple or bottle to use. They should be encouraged to bring their personal feeding equipment from home. However, many parents admit to having had to experiment with a variety of nipples before achieving some level of feeding success. The SLP, working with the medical/habilitative team, may also need to try an array of equipment options before arriving at a satisfactory choice. Morris and Klein (1987) provide descriptions of commercially available feeding equipment, including nipples. Their recommendations for identifying an effective nipple include the following:

- Avoid artificially enlarged holes that cause a rapid uncontrolled flow of liquid.
- Use nipples that fit the size and shape of the infant's mouth.
- Softer nipples may be more appropriate for the infant whose suck is weak or who tends to become fatigued easily. However, the nipple should not collapse with sucking.
- A nipple with a thin or narrowed area between the gums facilitates the infant who has a jaw thrust or a bite reflex.

Other items described by Morris and Klein (1987) include various types of pacifiers, bottles, cups, straws, and spoons. See Appendix B for descriptions of available equipment.

TIMING OF THERAPEUTIC INPUT

Timing of input depends on many variables. Generally, when an infant is medically stable, at least 34 weeks gestational age, and has demonstrated good weight gain, feeding begins. Many immature infants demonstrate "disorganized feeding." Disorganized feeding behaviors in NICU and PICU infants are characterized by problems with low energy levels, immature sucking, sucking disorganization, poor neurobehavioral control, and an immature oral-motor musculature. VandenBerg (1990) suggests these behaviors are frequently resolved through maturation and the incorporation of strategies by caregivers to foster neurobehavioral organization. Intervention with disorganized feeders should focus on assisting the infant in learning self-regulation of the autonomic, motor, and state systems described by Als (1982) before targeting oral-motor intervention.

When infants are medically stable, with adequate gastrointestinal functioning, but demonstrate dysfunctional feeding behaviors (abnormal muscle tone or very abnormal cheek, lip, jaw and tongue movements), speech-language intervention by a skilled therapist is needed. If feeding difficulties are not addressed early, the sick infant is put at a higher risk for poor growth and potentially, a longer course of hospitalization.

FEEDING PROBLEMS FREQUENTLY TARGETED BY THE SLP IN PICU INTERVENTION

Most infants referred for feeding consults demonstrate feeding behaviors characterized by emesis and gagging. Abnormal oral activity seen includes the tonic bite reflex, tongue retraction, jaw thrusting, tongue protrusion and the tongue locking against the roof of the mouth.

According to Alexander and Beecher (1992), "Most of what a child does during feeding is related to airway maintenance and/or airway protection." Therapeutic intervention may revolve around issues related to facilitating self-regulation, making environmental adaptations, positioning the child, choosing feeding equipment and handling techniques to normalize respiration and oral-motor muscle-tone. Other considerations may include the thickness, taste, and temperature of the foods presented. For children with respiratory problems who require oxygen supplementation, providing additional oxygen to reduce fatigue during feeding may also be considered by the feeding team.

There is no one simple approach for assisting all infants with feeding problems. Several suggestions follow that may facilitate feeding with some infants.

Positioning:

As indicated earlier in this chapter, positioning is an important aspect of any feeding program. Both the feeder and the infant must be in comfortable, well-supported positions. When providing intervention, the feeder holds or supports the child in a position which provides stability, maintenance of an open airway and appropriate body alignment. For many children at least three months of age (corrected for prematurity), the head is flexed forward in a chin tuck to facilitate normal swallowing. If the child is seated in a high chair or infant seat, pillow and/or towel rolls may be needed to maintain the child in the desired position. Feeding is a "flexor" skill and positioning should address that aspect. However, children who appear to use head extension as a way to maintain an open airway need further evaluation by way of oral-pharyngeal motiliity (video-swallow) studies to determine the optimal positioning for safe feeding.

Sucking:

Many infants grow fatigued easily during feeding and cease sucking. These infants may signal they need a break due to fatigue and/or loss of their suck-swallow-breathe rhythm. Intermittent rest periods should be provided. They may also be assisted by the provision of jaw and cheek stability. This is accomplished by pulling the cheeks forward and steadying the jaw. For infants who cannot maintain lip closure, the use of larger nipples and stabilization of their lower jaw while gently pushing up the lower lip may facilitate the feeding process. However, caution is needed, as mouth breathers will only tolerate brief moments of lip closure.

The SLP, occupational therapist and/or physical therapist frequently work together to inhibit abnormal oral reactions, to facilitate respiration, and to normalize oral-motor tone. To facilitate sucking, the SLP may use techniques involving the use of graded, deep pressure stimulation to the gums, lips, and tongue. As stated earlier, this input should not be provided until the child has learned to accept deep pressure stimulation to other parts of the body. Unanticipated input to the oral cavity is aversive to most individuals, no matter what age.

Tongue retraction:

Oral hypersensitivity is frequently characterized by tongue retraction upon introduction of the nipple. This is a common characteristic of neurologically impaired and/or stressed infants who have had prolonged periods of intubation, exposure to foul-tasting medications and other noxious oral experiences. Treatment usually involves handling techniques and positioning to promote oral relaxation. For some infants, prone shoulder-elevated positioning on the therapist's lap may help achieve the desired oral musculature outcome.

For others, the therapeutic technique of rapid tapping under the child's chin may inhibit tongue retraction. Input from an SLP is needed to determine the appropriate approach for each child.

Once an optimal position is achieved, and the tongue moves forward in a relaxed state, gradual introduction of stimulation (by finger glove, massage brush, toothbrush or bottle nipple) to the palate and the tongue is introduced. If tongue retraction suddenly reappears, stimulation should be withdrawn, and the infant should be aided in re-establishing neurobehavioral control before the stimulation is tried again.

Tongue protrusion

In neonates, reflexive suckling movements of the tongue frequently signal the mother that her child is hungry. Normally, this reflex can be elicited by touching the hungry infant's lips or cheek. It disappears in neurologically competent infants by age five months. Strong tongue protrusion or thrusting interferes with feeding at any age. However, infants with respiratory problems may use tongue protrusion as a means of alerting the feeder that they need an open airway and that they cannot achieve a suck-swallow-breathe pattern at that time. Those signs call for a brief rest period; the feeder should remove the feeding device from the oral cavity.

Once optimal positioning for maintenance of an open airway is determined by oral-pharyngeal motility (OPM) studies, one technique which may be used to inhibit tongue protrusion involves continuous rapid pushing down and back on the anterior portion of the tongue until the tongue draws back to the gum ridge. The bottle nipple, a Nuk brush, a rubber-tipped spoon, or your finger glove may be the instrument used. To avoid a bite reflex, do not place the instrument between and behind the gum ridges. If a bite reflex occurs, avoid pulling the object out of the mouth. Wait for the child's jaw to relax and drop before removing the item. Once the tongue recedes back, assist the infant in achieving lip closure on the spoon or cup. If sharp tongue retraction occurs and is maintained in a fixed position, this "pushing" technique may be inappropriate for that child.

Difficulty transitioning to new food textures

Normally, cereals and pureed foods are introduced into a child's diet by age four to six months. By the age of eight months, an infant accepts lumpier textures, such as junior foods and mashed table foods. By 12 months, an infant is introduced to chopped table foods and tolerates cup-drinking. By age 24 months, competent biting, chewing, cup-drinking and swallowing of most food textures and liquids has emerged. Each food transition stage is preceded by maturation of neuromotor and neurobehavioral controls. As infants gain more motor control, they expand in their capacity to experiment with new foods.

Neurologically involved youngsters frequently exhibit atypical neuromotor development and aberrant sensorimotor channels. Disordered taste, smell, sight, touch, and/or proprioception combined with motor-planning problems interfere with normal processing and handling of the sensory information provided by new foods.

Children with these disorders may respond to any new oral experience by gagging, vomiting and/or aspirating. If gastrointestinal functioning is adequate and swallowing is normal, an oral normalization program is called for. Initially, this is conducted by helping the child get her own hands to her mouth and by encouraging oral exploration of safe objects, e.g. toys, spoons. Once the child tolerates oral play, the therapist may gradually introduce new tastes and temperatures by means of washcloth, toys, or feeding utensils put to the child's lips and then on her gums. The therapist hopes to encourage new oral-motor responses, e.g., lip smacking, tongue lateralization, cheek movement, as well as a beginning acceptance of new stimulation.

Children with neuromotor sensory disorders have variable response patterns to tastes and temperatures. For very involved children, tart, salty tastes and/or cold temperatures may provide desired sensory feeding responses. Through experimentation, the caregiver needs to determine what the child prefers. Once acceptance is established for a new taste, e.g. pureed sweet potatoes, that food should be offered for several meals over several days before another new taste of the same texture is introduced. The caregiver should warmly reinforce, with smiles and kisses, all attempts by the infant to experiment with foods.

If a child has been identified as at risk for aspiration, choices in food textures are critical. Through use of video fluoroscopic oral-pharyngeal motility (OPM) studies, determination as to safe oral handling of various textures is determined. Children with severe neuromotor disorders and cognitive delays frequently cannot tolerate textures that exceed their functional developmental levels.

Feeding progress usually occurs if the caregivers are consistent in their approach and carefully share information with each other. Feeding progress may be slow, as frequent interruptions due to health setbacks occur in the chronically ill population.

Facilitating Teaming

The team meetings should provide an opportunity for professionals to reevaluate priorities, educate each other as to rationales for treatment approaches and determine how best to implement and monitor their use. Issues regarding the need for direct therapeutic intervention versus use of a consultative approach require ongoing discussion and agreement.

Once a treatment plan is developed by the team and a primary handler is identified, the clinician becomes responsible for closely monitoring the infant's responses, using chart review, observations and/or by weekly team meetings. This information must be logged and the treatment plan must regularly be reevaluated and revised.

All too often SLPs are not called on until the transition from tube to oral feeding in PICU infants is anticipated. By then, many infants have developed negative responding behaviors to oral-motor input. To assist medical caregivers in developing an awareness of the need for earlier intervention, information sharing sessions with early intervention providers should be scheduled. Giving presentations at interdisciplinary pediatric grand rounds and volunteering for unidisciplinary in-service training sessions (e.g., nursing, dietary, occupational therapy, physical therapy, or child-life) are vehicles for information dissemination. Providing families and staff with appropriate reading materials and handouts regarding oral normalization approaches prompts helpful discussion and builds understanding.

The infant development specialist and other caregivers can integrate suggestions from the SLP into their daily routines with each infant. When personal contact with the child's parents is not possible, a written log with illustrations may be used to keep them updated on feeding techniques, intervention strategies, and their infant's responses. Parents should be encouraged to use the same log to make comments, ask questions, and report on their observations.

Daily or weekly treatment goals and objectives may be attached to each child's isolette or bed. Written directions with pictures are an effective means of encouraging follow-up by busy hospital staff. A daily visit to each infant is beneficial, as children are frequently reassigned to different rooms or different wards as their status changes. When this happens, treatment plans may inadvertently be lost and need replacing. New staff require orientation in each child's treatment regimen. Staff input regarding necessary treatment revisions should be elicited. Experienced nursing staff are able to offer creative and effective ideas for enhancing oral-motor function and increasing nutrient intake by mouth.

A carefully conceived treatment plan, which is supported by the infant's family and the medical/habilitative team, has a high chance for success. Patience, flexibility, and cooperation of all team members are essential ingredients to any habilitative care plan. Chronic feeding problems require a long-term therapeutic program and frequent modifications. Open communication lines among all team members ensure program consistency.

REFERENCES

Alexander, R. & Beecher, R. (1992, March.) Pediatric Oral-Pharyngeal (Video-swallow) Studies. Presented by Memorial Hospital Pediatric Rehabilitation Services, Colorado Springs, CO.

Alexander, R. (1983). Developing pre-speech and feeding abilities in children. In S. Shanks (Ed.), *Nursing and the management of pediatric communication disorders*, 165-223. San Diego: College Hill Press.

Als, H. (1982). Toward a synactive theory of development: Promise for the assessment and support of infant individuality. *Infant Mental Health Journal.* 3(4), 229-243.

Behrman, M.M., Jones, J.K., & Wilds, M.L. (1989). Technology intervention with very young children with disabilities. *Infants and Young Children*, 1(4), 66-77.

Bess, F.H., Peck, B.F., & Chapman, J.J. (1979). Further observations on noise levels in infant incubators. *Pediatrics,* 63(1): 100-106.

Braun, M. & Palmer, M.M. (1982). *Early detection and treatment of the infant and young child with neuromuscular disorders.* New York: Therapeutic Media.

Brinker, R., & Lewis, M. (1982). Making the world work with microcomputers: A learning prosthesis for handicapped infants. *Exceptional Child*, 49(2): 163-170.

Chatoor, I. (1991, December). *Assessment of feeding interaction. Presented at special interest session Failure-to-thrive: A national multidisciplinary perspective.* National Center for Clinical Infant Programs Seventh Biennial Training Institute. Washington, DC.

Crane, L.D. (1986). Cardiorespiratory management of the high risk neonate: Implications for developmental therapists. In J.K. Sweeney (Ed.), *The high risk neonate: Developmental therapy perspectives.* New York: Haworth Press. 255-279.

Goldberger, J. & Wolfer, J. (1991). An approach for identifying potential threats to development in hospitalized toddlers. *Infants and Young Children*, 3(3), 74-83.

Gorski, P.A., Davison, M.F., & Brazelton, T.B. (1979). Stages of behavioral organization in the high risk neonate: Theoretical and clinical considerations. *Seminars in Perinatology*, 3(1), 61-72.

Gottfried, A.W., Lande, P.W, Brown, S.S., King, J., Coen, C.V. & Hodgman, J.E. (1981). Physical and social environment of newborn infants in special care units. *Science,* 214: 673-675.

Goudreau, A.L., Whan, M.Q., Stelmachowicz, P.G., & Wallace, K.L. (1989, November). *Relevant factors in the identification of hearing loss.* Presented at the American Speech-Language-Hearing Association Convention, St. Louis, MO.

Harris, M.B. (1986). Oral-motor management of the high risk infant. In J.K. Sweeney, (Ed.), *The high risk neonate: developmental therapy perspectives.* New York: Haworth Press. 231-251.

Imhoff, S.M. & Wigginton, V.M. (1991). Identifying feeding and swallowing problems in infants and young children. *Clinics in Communication Disorders,* 1(2), 59-68.

Joint Committee on Infant Hearing. (1991). 1990 position statement. ASHA (American Speech-Language-Hearing Association) , 33 (Suppl. 5), 3-6.

Kamen, R.S. & Watson, B.C. (1991). Effects of long term tracheostomy on spectral characteristics of vowel production. *Journal of Speech and Hearing Research,* 34: 1057-1065.

Karchmer, M.A. (1985). A demographic perspective. In E. Cherow, N.D. Matkin, & R.J. Trybus (Eds.), *Hearing-impaired children and youth with disabilities.* Washington, DC: Gallaudet Press.

Moore, M.C. & Green, H.L. (1985). Tube feeding of infants and children. Pediatric Clinics of North America, 32(2), 401-417.

Morris, S E. & Klein, M.D. (1987). *Pre-feeding skills.* Tucson: Therapy Skill Builders. 312-313.

Palmer, M. (1989). *Feeding problems and treatment strategies for infants with BPD, drug addiction, tracheostomies, and neuromuscular disorders.* Presented at Contemporary Forums Conference: Developmental Interventions in Neonatal Care, New Orleans, LA.

VandenBerg, K.A. (1990). Nippling management of the sick neonate in the NICU: The disorganized feeder. *Neonatal Network,* 9(1), 9-16.

Chapter 6

Service Coordination and Chronically Ill Infants

Kathy S. Katz, Ph.D.

The complexities of identifying and addressing the needs of chronically ill young children require close coordination of intervention personnel. In recent years, the approach in providing interdisciplinary services to children with disabilities has been to designate one professional as a "service coordinator." This individual assumes the responsibility of working with the family to coordinate the assessment of the child and to assist them in securing the needed services identified by the assessment process.

The concept of the service coordinator role has been included as part of federal legislation that assures early intervention services for children from birth to three, Public Law 99-457, recently updated as IDEA Part H. Under the legislation, one of the professionals providing services to the child and family is assigned the role of service coordinator or shares this role jointly with the family itself. This role may be referred to by a number of terms, including "case manager" and "care coordinator," among others. All terms refer to an individual who is intended to serve as a major support to families in securing the myriad of services needed by a child with complex medical and developmental problems.

The overall role to be provided by a service coordinator includes:

- Coordinating the assessment process
- Participating in the development of an Individualized Family Service Plan (IFSP)
- Assisting the family in identifying and accessing appropriate services
- Coordinating and monitoring services
- Facilitating program transitions.

(Bailey, 1989).

ASSIGNMENT OF THE SERVICE COORDINATOR

Much discussion has occurred in recent years as to what disciplinary background is best suited for assuming the role of service coordinator. Some early interventionists have argued that because a wide *knowledge of community resources* is necessary in implementing early intervention plans, social workers and nurse specialists are best suited to be service coordinators since they have the greatest knowledge in this area. Others have argued that a member of the discipline that deals with *the child's greatest area of disability* will have the most relevant knowledge for implementing an intervention plan. A third argument is that a *professional discipline of service coordinator* with individuals specifically trained to handle responsibilities of service coordination is the most effective solution and will provide the most objective support to families (Bailey, 1989).

In the hospital setting, the service coordinator may fill the additional role of advocate for the family in helping to clarify medical concerns. Additionally, the hospital-based service coordinator may serve as a liaison with the community, helping to identify the variety of support services necessary for the child to be cared for in the home.

This chapter will discuss the activities involved in service coordination for families of chronically ill children, especially in regards to discharge planning and development of the IFSP.

INITIAL CONTACTS

Once a family has been identified as appropriate for early intervention services in the hospital, a service coordinator is designated. The decision as to whom to designate may be based on one of two premises. The first is to utilize a random rotation of team members, with each of them trained to handle these particular responsibilities. This approach follows a transdisciplinary format in that the service coordinator will draw on other team members for guidance in assisting the family in accessing resources.

A second approach is to select an individual from the discipline that is related to the child's major disability area as the service coordinator. An example illustrating this approach is a situation with a child who has a major motor disability. This child and family may be served best by a service coordinator with a background in physical therapy. A service coordinator with particular expertise in the area of the primary disability may provide the best support to families in terms of identifying and accessing the most appropriate resources for the family and the infant.

The designated service coordinator confirms the attending physician's approval of the child's involvement. The service coordinator, through notes, phone contact or direct contact with the family, arranges a time and place that will be convenient for them to meet together. The service coordinator might make the initial contact with either parent, whoever is at the hospital on a particular day, and set a time to meet with both parents, if possible, at a subsequent date. The initial contact provides an opportunity to explain the intervention program procedures to the parents and to ascertain the parents' readiness for involvement. At a very acute phase of their child's illness, the parents may not be emotionally prepared to consider nonmedical issues. For other families, being able to look at the healthy aspects of their child in terms of development may provide an avenue for them to play a special role in their child's care plan. It is important for the service coordinator to be sensitive to whether the introduction of an intervention program is timely.

The attending physician and child's nurse may be helpful in preparing the family to consider involvement in intervention. Obtaining the physician's approval is essential before any overture is made to the family.

DEVELOPING THE ASSESSMENT PLAN

Once the service coordinator has met with the family, and they have agreed to be involved in intervention, planning for the assessment may begin. While in the past professionals usually made independent decisions about what the diagnostic issues were and often employed a standard battery of measures to assess them, the assessment process with young children today must be responsive to family concerns.

The service coordinator begins by exploring with the family the particular questions or concerns they have about their **child's development or care needs**. Parents often have concerns about their child's motor development or language development, as these areas are typically delayed in chronically ill children. Families may also have concerns about a particular area of health management.

The service coordinator reviews these concerns with the family and suggests possible strategies for assessing those problems. The service coordinator may need time to review the concerns with other team members to get their ideas as to recommended approaches for evaluation of that issue.

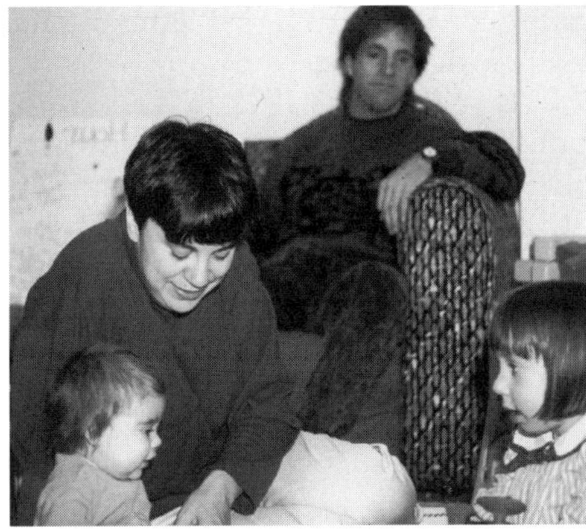

While the goal for assessment in the family-centered approach is that the parents will determine what areas will be assessed, it is important for professionals to provide them adequate information on which to base their decisions in this regard. For instance, a family may express their chief concern as their child's lack of speech. Their preference for the assessment, then, is to evaluate receptive and expressive language. This same family may not have a particular concern about their child's intellectual functioning and might not see the necessity of IQ testing. The service coordinator can assist the family by explaining that to gain a better understanding of their child's current capability for language, they can get an important piece of information from an overall cognitive assessment.

In fact, IDEA Part H requires a statement of the child's current functioning in the areas of physical development, cognitive development, communication development, social-emotional development and adaptive development as part of the IFSP process. This part of the assessment process will be most familiar to professionals. For chronically ill children, the assessment process should also include information on the child's medical condition that may make an impact on development.

As a further part of assessment planning, the family's desires for their child and the family as a whole must be delineated. In an effort to have the parents' goals for their child be meaningful in a real world context, it is helpful if these goals are expressed in functional terms and reflect the individual family's priorities for their child. Rather than expressing the concern as, "Why doesn't my child talk?", this goal could be stated as, "I would like my child to be able to communicate his needs at the dinner table."

As a final part of planning the assessment, the parents' preferences for their own involvement in the test sessions must be ascertained. Some parents will choose to be present during assessment. Other families may feel that their child will perform better if they are not present. Since parents generally have good ability to predict their child's performance, their suggestions should be included in planning the assessment procedures.

If the child has previously been involved in an early intervention program or in a high risk infant follow-up program, information from these programs should be obtained. If the child's health was more stable at the time of the previous assessment, that assessment may serve as a baseline measure in considering the reliability of assessment findings during hospitalization. On the other hand, the child's current abilities need to be considered in terms of program planning during the hospitalization.

While **family assessment** may be an important avenue for information gathering for the development of an IFSP, this type of family assessment is not meant to be intrusive or judgmental (McGonigel and Garland, 1988). This means that the process is quite different from that which has been used in family assessment in mental health consultation. This latter approach has tended to focus on psychopathology in family functioning.

As part of the IFSP process, information is provided voluntarily by the family about those areas of family life which are relevant to the child's development (McGonigel et al. 1991). The family makes the determination about what is relevant. If they choose not to elect a family assessment, this is acceptable under IDEA Part H. In terms of discharge planning for a medically fragile infant, however, some determination must be made of the family's ability to manage medical needs in the home setting. Some aspects of the voluntary nature of the information gathering process thus differ somewhat when major health issues must be considered.

Determination of the child's functioning in the major developmental areas is achieved through use of a variety of assessment tools and strategies. These are described in Chapter 4.

Assessment of Family Needs

Information gathering in relation to needs identified by the family may be achieved through a number of sources. Open discussion between the service coordinator and the family is a major avenue. Use of written surveys and checklists may also provide a structured means for helping families define areas of need.

The information gathered by interview should be considered an evolving process that will probably begin with the first contact between the service coordinator and the family. This process continues even after the development of a formal IFSP, making it a responsive, working document.

At all times, the information provided by families must be considered confidential and information should not be shared without permission from the family. Team members must be sensitive in maintaining family confidences, even in informal discussions with each other (McGonigel et al., 1991).

The following principles taken from McGonigel et al. (1991) should guide the process for identifying the family's concerns, priorities, and resources:

- The inclusion of family information in the IFSP is voluntary on the part of families.
- The identification of family concerns, priorities, and resources is based on an individual family's determination of which aspects of family life are relevant to the child's development.
- A family need or concern exists only if the family perceives that the need or concern exists.
- Families have a broad array of formal and informal options to choose from in determining how they will identify their concerns, priorities, and resources.
- Families have multiple and continuing opportunities to identify their concerns, priorities, and resources.
- Family confidences are respected, and family-shared information is not discussed casually among staff.
- The process of identifying family concerns, priorities and resources leads to the development of IFSP outcomes, strategies, and activities that help families achieve the things they want from early intervention for their children and themselves.

Structured Surveys of Family Needs

Families of a child newly identified as having special needs may not be aware of the variety of resources that are available to enhance their child's development. They may not have even thought about the areas of knowledge in which they would like more information. Use of structured surveys of family needs are especially helpful to these families . These surveys have been developed by early interventionists based on those areas of need that are typically expressed by families of children with disabilities.

These surveys typically outline needs for information, support, ways to explain to others, finances, available community services and family functioning. Some of the surveys also provide suggestions for areas in which the family can identify its current strengths and resources, which is an equally important part of the IFSP development. Some of the major questionnaires used for needs surveys include:

- Family Needs Survey, Revised Edition (Bailey & Simeonsson, 1990)
- Family Needs Scale (Dunst et al., 1988)
- Family Support Scale (Dunst et al., 1988)
- Carolina Parent Support Scale (Bristol, 1983)
- Parent Needs Survey (Seligman & Benjamin-Darling, 1989)

While these surveys provide a great deal of information about the family and community service needs, they are limited in regard to needs a family may have in managing a child with complex medical problems. In an effort to develop a survey that would include areas of needs related to medical management, a "Survey for Families of Children with Special Health Care Needs" was developed through Project Headed Home of the Georgetown University Child Development Center that was a combined adaptation of the *Family Needs Survey* of Bailey & Simeonsson (1985) and the *Needs for Home Care* (Kaufman & Lichtenstein). This survey appears in Appendix C. The service coordinator reviews the responses provided by the family on the survey to learn what areas to explore and expand upon through the family interview.

Additionally, "Managing my Child's Medical Needs," another questionnaire developed for Project Headed Home, provides more specific information on parent training needs in respect to specific medical problems of the child. (See Appendix D.)

Family Interviews

In the preparation of early intervention service providers across professional disciplines, it has become increasingly important to include training in interviewing skills. One of the major principles in family interviews for the purpose of IFSP development is that the family take the lead in identifying areas of concern. The early interventionist facilitating the discussion must assume the role of an active listener who helps to clarify and cluster the major areas of need voiced by the family in expressing their concerns.

Active listening should include the following points identified by Turnbull et al. (1991):

a. Listen for cultural and family values that are important to the family.
b. Listen for the names of family members, friends, and professionals who are already in the support network and whose support has been particularly valued.
c. Listen for interests, needs, and strengths that might link the child and family with a wider network of supporters.
d. Listen for the coping strategies that the family uses and any expressed desire for expanding coping strategies.

e. Listen for things that the family would like to do to help their child and to help themselves (To Do list).
f. Listen for how the family has typically approached solving problems in the past.
g. Listen for the concerns, hopes, and plans that the family has concerning transitional issues.
h. Listen for the kinds of evaluations that have been conducted in the past and the evaluation questions that they would like to have addressed.
i. Listen for and acknowledge the specific strengths the family has shown in adjusting to their child's disability in meeting the child's needs.

For hospitalized children, the information gathered up to this point may be consolidated into a number of areas of strengths and needs that should be addressed during the hospitalization. This is especially important in terms of the needs the family may have identified in respect to involvement in the child's caregiving during his hospitalization and in needs for training in specific medical management procedures prior to discharge.

The service coordinator reviews the findings of the various professionals assessing the child and the needs identified by the family. These are then organized into areas for discussion with the family to formulate an **interim intervention plan**, especially designed toward promoting readiness for discharge. The interim plan is continually modified during the hospitalization through the collaboration of the family, the service coordinator, the developmental team, and medical/nursing caregivers. Modifications generally reflect the changing medical status of the child and the family's confidence and competence in self-management of medical caregiving needs.

When it is anticipated that the child will require prolonged hospitalization, rather than develop an interim plan, the service coordinator and the family may elect to formulate a formal IFSP. In some states this may be done in conjunction with local early intervention administrative agencies responsible for child-find activities. The family may thus be eligible for various developmental support services even though their child remains hospitalized. The procedure for development of the IFSP will be discussed later in this chapter. The actual procedure for developing an IFSP will not differ greatly if it is done during hospitalization or at discharge.

Service Coordinator Function during Hospitalization

The service coordinator attempts to **maintain frequent contact with the family** throughout the hospitalization. This may require evening visits to the ward and frequent phone contact. Maintaining a communication book may help facilitate the exchange of information among family, service coordinator, and medical staff.

The service coordinator also assumes a primary role in providing **consultation to nurses** caring for the child, focusing on developmental needs of the child and the overall family needs. The service coordinator demonstrates developmental activities that can be integrated into caregiving routines to the nurses and responds to questions they may have. In some instances, the service coordinator may assist the family in having particular medical or nursing recommendations clarified when the family has questions about them.

The service coordinator may, in many instances, also be a direct service provider, working directly with the child on the goals of the intervention plan. **Regular team meetings**, at which the service coordinator updates the developmental team on current needs of the child and family, is the primary means for continued team input.

One of the most active periods for the service coordinator will be during preparation for discharge. This is, in fact, an ongoing process. The service coordinator continues to work with the family to identify needs that must be met if the child is to be managed in the home setting.

ACTIVITIES IN PREPARATION FOR DISCHARGE

Discharge planning for medically fragile children will require assessment of several major areas that will impact on the child's daily care. These include the following:

- Parents' medical self-management skills
- Physical home environment for caring for a child with chronic health care needs
- Necessary community support services

Family's Medical Caregiving Skills

The issue of determining the family's level of competence in medical caregiving procedures is an important one because training in this area may be implemented immediately after admission and an ongoing training plan may be developed.

While the medical/nursing staff will assume a large part of the responsibility for training families to provide medical caregiving to their infants, the developmental team can provide additional support and training for families. One means for assessing the family comfort level in performing medical caregiving routines is through a survey such as "Managing my Child's Medical Needs," shown in Appendix D. This questionnaire may be given to families at the time that the child and family assessment measures are gathered. Areas of caregiving needs with which the parents are not comfortable can thus be identified. Collaborative decisions can be made on the goals to be set that will help the parents develop confidence in particular skills.

The child's nurse will usually work closely with the family in practicing medical caregiving routines. It may be valuable for the service coordinator or developmental team nurse to participate in some of these sessions so they may continue to provide assistance and support to families as they master new skills.

Assessment of the Physical Home Environment

When a child will be discharged home still dependent on medical technological equipment, the assessment of the home environment will be particularly important in determining its adequacy for support of the equipment. A number of assessment questionnaires have been developed to assist with this task, and they are described by Katz et al. (1989).

In general, it must be determined if there is sufficient space in the home for the equipment. The adequacy of things such as the electrical supply must also be evaluated if the medical equipment requires specific levels. These needs must be identified in adequate time if any reconstruction will be necessary prior to discharge.

Community Support Needs

This represents the largest area for which assessment and planning will be required. In terms of meeting the infant's medical needs, community supports may include:

- A variety of vendors who provide medical equipment or supplies
- Agencies that provide home nursing care

- Emergency medical services
- Sources for pharmacy supplies
- Developmental and social support services

At a point several weeks ahead of what might be the anticipated discharge date, a discharge planning conference should be called. Those participating at the conference generally will be the following:

- The family
- Medical specialists
- Primary nurses
- Service Coordinator
- Attending physician
- Social worker

At this meeting, information gathered from the assessment will be reviewed with the family and a list of discharge needs will be formulated. The responsibilities for providing training in an area or exploring community resources will be divided up among members of the team and a time line for completion of those tasks will be set.

After this meeting, the family will be encouraged to take on increasing amounts of the child's caregiving needs, with nursing guidance close at hand. The developmental team will continue to look for ways that developmental goals and activities might be integrated into caregiving routines. They will also provide guidance to the family in carrying them out.

The primary nurse, or sometimes a specifically designated discharge nurse, will continue to review the progress in moving towards readiness for discharge in terms of parent training and community service supports. A social worker associated with the PICU may also assume some of the responsibility in coordinating the community-based health supports. Usually a few days before discharge another meeting will be called to review the final discharge plan.

Once at home, a variety of levels of nursing support may be available to the family. Some children will require many hours of skilled nursing during the day, and the parent may not assume the major responsibility for direct medical caregiving. For other families, visiting nurses or public health nurses may be available to ease the transition to home management through weekly or sometimes daily visits.

In an ideal circumstance, a nurse, familiar to the family from the hospital where the child was cared for, might make several home visits in the immediate post-discharge period. The service coordinator may also play a supportive role by meeting with the family at home after discharge. Again, the service coordinator may help the family find answers to questions they have about the child's care. Once the family has had the child at home a week or two, the needs they identified for themselves will be realistic in terms of the child's ongoing management needs. This is a good time for the service coordinator to move ahead with the formal IFSP process, possibly in conjunction with a representative from the community-based early intervention agency.

The Family-Centered Interview

In the past, when an intervention plan was developed, it was usually formulated by professionals, independent of the family. The family were receivers of the recommended plan, often without having an opportunity to provide input of their own. Under current mandates of IDEA Part H, the family's relationship with professionals

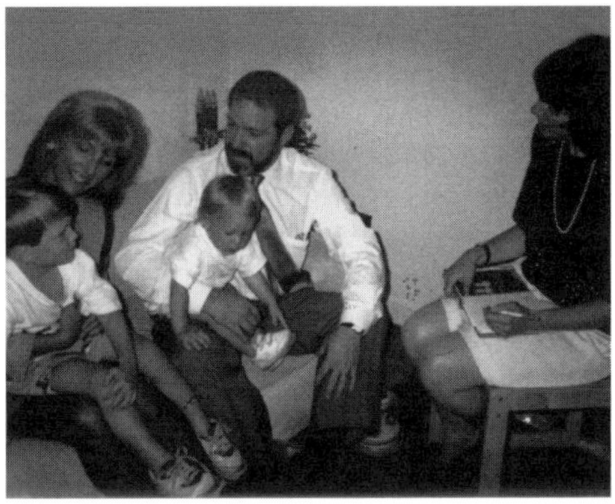

and their involvement in the development of the IFSP follows an entirely new philosophy. It is family members themselves who:

- Identify their own strengths and needs
- Decide on the intervention goals
- Determine the relative importance of each of these goals

The family's determination of their strengths and needs is done in collaboration with the interdisciplinary team through interviews and formal assessment. The service coordinator assists by organizing the information gathered during the assessment into several groupings that form the basis of discussion of strengths and needs in the **family-centered interview** (Winton & Bailey, 1988).

The interview is intended to be an open-ended forum through which the service plan can be sketched. It is best held where the family feels most comfortable, often in their home. The family should choose who should participate as family representatives. They may choose to include extended family members or particular friends who are involved with the child in special needs or who play an important support role for the family.

The role of the service coordinator is to serve as a *facilitator* of the discussion, but not to direct the discussion. The role of the service coordinator, as well as other professionals working with the family, will require the following skills described by Bailey (1987):

- To look at families from a systems perspective
- To identify relevant family needs
- To use appropriate testing and interviewing techniques
- To negotiate with families to reach joint solutions
- To help families match their needs with available resources in their community

Some professionals will require practice to develop family interviewing techniques. They may accomplish this through role playing sessions.

Upon meeting with the family, the service coordinator introduces the format by which the interview will be conducted. The structure for the interview usually includes the following:

a) Introduction
b) Delineation of family strengths
c) Identification of family needs
d) Formulation of functional outcomes
e) Establishment of priority of goals
f) Determination of activities to achieve goals, time line for implementation, and person /persons responsible for overseeing each activity
g) Summary, finalization of plan, and review date set
h) Conclusion

The service coordinator can facilitate the meeting at the beginning by reviewing the format, reassuring the family about confidentiality, establishing a general time frame for the discussion, and making it clear that he or she will guide but not direct the discussion.

Discussing **family strengths** is a good way to begin. In the case of a child with chronic illness, the focus has often been on the child's problems and on the family's need for assistance. Both professionals and families themselves can build a more balanced perspective of family needs if the strengths and resources of a family and child are recognized as well. The family will usually be able to describe several strengths that they see in themselves and their child. The service coordinator may be able to add some additional resources identified by the family assessment process.

In moving on to discuss **family concerns**, it may be helpful for the service coordinator to pose several areas for discussion that may link some of the needs stated by the family in responses to the assessment measures. For instance, the service coordinator might have identified three major areas:

1) Need for financial assistance
2) Need for alternative child care resources
3) Need for more information about the child's medical status

Within these major areas, several specific needs may have been expressed during the assessment phase and could be expanded upon during the family interview. Once all the current needs have been elicited, the family may begin to organize these according to their relative importance. The next step is to express the needs in terms of **functional outcomes** or goals. For example, rather than say that the child has a need for language intervention, the goal might be stated as, "Julie will be able to indicate when she is hungry or thirsty to her caregivers." Once the desired outcome has been described, the activities for achieving it are listed. For the above example, the activities might be described as follows:

- Individual sessions with the speech pathologist, focusing on communicating needs
- A home program designed by the speech pathologist for the parents to encourage Julie to communicate at home
- Consultation to the early intervention classroom teacher by the speech pathologist to carry over communication goals

Additionally, the **individual/or individuals responsible** for implementing and monitoring that activity are designated. A **time line** that indicates the start date and duration of the activity should also be included.

After the plan for each of the functional outcomes desired by the family has been developed, a date is set for evaluating the progress made in meeting the goals.

The service coordinator then reviews with the family the plan that has been outlined and incorporates any changes they want to make. The session is then concluded with an agreement to reconvene at the time determined.

The key to an effective IFSP is collaborative goal setting by the team of parents and professionals. It may be that the family does not see as a priority a desirable outcome identified by a professional. Although the ultimate decision is up to the family, the professionals should feel free to communicate their own recommendations. The communication and clarification of the professionals' judgment will help the family to make an informed decision. A sample IFSP appears in Appendix E.

After the list of activities or services needed for the desired outcomes has been completed, the service coordinator, along with other individuals identified in the plan, assists the family in obtaining these services. To accomplish this may require the service coordinator to contact the necessary agencies directly or to provide the family with contact information.

Revisions should be made in the final IFSP as needed. A full reevaluation of progress is usually made at six-month to one-year intervals. Evaluation of progress is usually made by rating each of the outcomes as successfully completed or to what degree progress has been achieved. Goal attainment rating scales have been developed by Bailey, et al. (1986) and Dunst et al.(1988).

For chronically ill children, the IFSP will probably include a variety of health-related as well as developmental and family support outcomes. The number of community services required by the child while in home care is extensive. The service coordinator plays an important role in coordinating these services. At the same time, it is important for the family to be advocating for their own child and developing the skills necessary for getting community agencies to respond to identified needs. Because the family will be the ongoing decision-maker and change agent for the child, it is important for them to play an active role in advocating for their child both before and after discharge from the hospital.

The responsibility of serving as service coordinator may shift as a child's age or circumstances change. While a chronically ill child may first have needed service coordination handled by hospital-based staff, once the child is enrolled in a community-based early intervention program, it may be preferable for a person from that agency to assume leadership in the development and revision of the IFSP. While the child continues to have prominent medical needs and frequent hospitalizations, continued service coordination by a hospital staff member will probably be necessary. The overall goal in service coordination and IFSP formulation for the chronically ill child is to provide support necessary for the family to normalize that child's experience as much as possible. For many children, this will mean being able to live at home with their families. For this to be achieved, however, requires the collaboration and coordination of a variety of professionals, agencies, and the family. It is a difficult goal to achieve but a very worthwhile one.

REFERENCES

Bailey, D. & Simeonsson, R. (1985). *The Family Needs Survey*. Chapel Hill, NC: Frank Porter Graham Child Development Center.

Bailey, D. & Simeonsson, R. (1990). *The Family Needs Survey-Revised*. Chapel Hill, NC: Frank Porter Graham Child Development Center.

Bailey, D. (1987). Collaborative goal setting with families: Resolving differences in values and priorities for services. *Topics in Early Childhood Special Education* 7(2), 59-71.

Bailey, D. (1989). Case management in early intervention. *Journal of Early Intervention*, 13,120-134.

Bailey, D., Simeonsson, R., Winton, P., Huntington, G., Comfort, M., Isbell, P., O'Donnell, K., & Helm, J. (1986). Family focused intervention: A functional model for planning, implementing and evaluating family services in early intervention. *Journal of the Division of Early Childhood* 10(2), 156-171.

Bristol, M. (1983). *Carolina Parent Support Scale*. Chapel Hill, NC: Frank Porter Graham Child Development Center.

Deal, A., Dunst, C., & Trivette, C. (1989). A flexible and functional approach to developing Individual Family Support Plans. *Infants and Young Children* 1(4), 32-43.

Dunst, C., Trivette, C. & Deal, A. (1988). *Enabling and empowering families: Principles and guidelines for practice.* Cambridge, MA: Brookline Books.

Katz, K., Pokorni, J., & Long, T. (1989) *Chronically ill and at risk infants: Family-centered intervention from hospital to home.* Palo Alto, CA: VORT Corp.

Kaufman, J. & Lichtenstein, K.A. *The family as service coordinator: Home care coordination for medically fragile children.* Washington, DC: Georgetown University Child Development Center.

McGonigel, M. & Garland, C. (1988). The Individualized Family Service Plan and the early intervention team: Team and family issues and recommended practices. *Infants and Young Children* 1(1), 10-21.

McGonigel, M., Kaufmann, R., & Johnson, B. (1991). *Guidelines and recommended practices for the Individualized Family Service Plan* (2nd ed.). Bethesda, MD: Association for the Care of Children's Health.

Seligman, M. & Benjamin-Darling, R. (1989). *Ordinary families, special children: A systems approach to childhood disability.* NY: Guilford Press.

Turnbull, A., Lee, I., & Turbiville, V. (1991). *IFSP Process Model.* Unpublished manuscript, University of Kansas, Beach Center on Families and Disability.

Winton, P. & Bailey, D. (1988). The family-focused interview: A collaborative mechanism for family assessment and goal setting. *Journal of the Division of Early Childhood* 12, 195-207.

Chapter 7

Providing Support to Families of Chronically Ill Children

Kathy S. Katz, Ph.D. and Deborah Powell Osborn, RN, Ed.M.

Early intervention for chronically ill children began in the 1950's in conjunction with the increasing capability to save premature infants through assisted ventilation. The early focus was on providing cognitive stimulation that theoretically was felt lacking in the NICU environment. These early investigations provided increased handling of the infants and enriched visual stimulation to compensate for the infants' purported lack of sensory experiences. The intervention was strictly infant-focused. Groups of infants in the NICU who received extra handling and stimulation were compared with other groups who did not receive the intervention. In fact, this type of intervention was successful in improving weight gain and reducing oxygen needs. However, these developmental advantages were lost after discharge. (Bennett, 1987).

In an effort to prolong the effectiveness of early intervention, theory shifted in the 1970's to focus on mother-child interaction as the target of early intervention. With this approach, the intent was to optimize the mother-child relationship by educating the mother in stimulation techniques. It was hoped that a more sustained effect of intervention would be seen if the mother were able to continue to employ stimulation strategies after discharge.

This shift in early intervention philosophy corresponded with studies of early intervention effectiveness with disadvantaged populations. Studies in the 1970's began to suggest that focus on the child alone through group intervention was not as effective if parents (usually mothers) were not involved in the program. Parent involvement began to be seen as a necessary part of early intervention (Bryant & Ramey, 1987).

In the later 1980's, with a greater appreciation for family systems theory, the target of early intervention for children who present with biological risks has focused on the family as a unit. The child is viewed within the context of his family and, for intervention to be effective, change must be directed at the unit as a whole. The notion of needing to address the family as a system goes one step further in recognizing that the family is a part of a larger social system often with competing demands. Intervention is designed not only to enhance development in the child but also to promote adaptive family functioning, furthering child development benefits (Bailey et al., 1986).

The 1980's brought a change in philosophy to early intervention by placing a new emphasis on parent-professional collaboration. The shift has been from the family as a passive receiver of services to its playing an active role as an equal in determining intervention goals and strategies.

For families of chronically ill children, this last decade has been marked by a tremendous change in medical management approaches for these children. Largely as a result of parent advocacy, chronically ill and technology-dependent children are now receiving home-based care in greater numbers. Previously, these children would have remained in acute care hospitals or intermediate care settings. With a complex network of community supports, families are now able to provide care for their chronically ill child within the context of the family.

Hospital-based intervention professionals can play an important role in providing the support needed by these families to enable them to assume the responsibility of home-based care. This discussion will explore some of the major issues with which families of children with complex medical needs must deal and for which professional support may be beneficial. While areas of need around which many families of chronically ill children may experience stress will be described, it is essential for intervention professionals to recognize that each family is unique. No two families will react identically to similar situations. One of the major goals in providing support to these families is to appreciate and capitalize upon particular coping strategies of a family as a whole and of individuals within the family.

HOSPITALIZATION FOR ACUTE ILLNESS

Most families experience their greatest degree of stress when their infant is acutely ill. The child's medical fragility is most apparent at these times, and the possibility of the child's death may be very real. A family's coping strategy may involve a need for a great deal of information from professionals, a need to talk with someone who is familiar with the child during periods of stable health, or a need for privacy. The interventionist must sensitively identify the needs of a particular family at that time. This may be achieved by asking the family directly or offering several options and seeing which the family selects.

Many families have described a need to feel that they have *control over certain decisions* at a time when most major health decisions are in the hands of the physicians. For these families, giving them some choices in roles they may play may be helpful in providing them some sense of control. Choices may revolve around such things as how and by whom a particular child caregiving activity will be carried out.

Families are often stressed by the rigid, somewhat arbitrary, and usually impersonal hospital policy rules. *Allowing flexibility in usual procedures* may make a big difference in not further exacerbating the stress a family experiences. Flexibility in such things as rooming in with the child or being able to assist or at least be present during an uncomfortable medical procedure will help the family see the institution as responsive to their situation.

Families will often have problems during hospitalization around *competing needs*. Guidance and support from professionals can assist them in finding solutions to reduce these needs. Examples would be needs for alternate caregivers for siblings of the ill child or transportation needs to the hospital.

Availability of *peer support* may greatly enhance the support provided by professionals. A parent "drop in" hour on the ward can provide parents with an opportunity to share experiences with other families facing similar stresses. A social service professional may serve as a facilitator at this session without necessarily directing discussion. The legitimacy of a family who has lived through a particular experience will have great relevance to a family seeking coping strategies. Other families will often share community supports they have discovered which may not be known to the hospital staff, thus expanding the community resource database that many hospitals try to maintain.

Attempts to *normalize routines* should be made in caregiving activities. The family should be provided an opportunity to describe how routines are handled at home, and when possible, the parent should be encouraged to perform the routine as it is usually done at home. If the child wears her hair a certain way, or uses a particular spoon for eating, these routines can be carried over into the hospital care plan, often despite acute illness. Familiar routines may reduce stress for the child herself but may also reassure families that their children are viewed as individuals.

Needs for information and regular communication with the medical/nursing care providers are two additional areas in which the interventionist may support the family in expressing their needs in this regard. The primary nurse is usually a good source of information, and both the family and the interventionist should maintain regular contact with him or her. Medical personnel are often very busy and their day-to-day communication may be brief. Most try to be responsive, however, to a family's need for a more expanded discussion.

Formal counseling may be a support needed by families as they struggle to cope with a medical crisis for their child. Most hospitals have a social worker responsible for service to the intensive care unit, who is often available to provide crisis intervention counseling to parents. A psychiatrist or psychologist with particular interest in working with chronic illness issues may be available within the hospital to meet with the family. A family may have selected a particular staff member as their preferred support person who does not have a background in provision of psychotherapeutic intervention. When this is the situation and a family may seem in need of more formal counseling, the interventionist may sensitively suggest to the family the availability of this additional support. This is not to suggest that the interventionist should withdraw from the role of support provider in that this less formal support may continue to be of benefit to the family.

The acute illness period is one often described by parents as a roller coaster. One day the child may appear to be on the road to recovery, only to have a major setback occur. Sometimes just being with a family in the evening hours during a crisis will make apparent the interventionist's commitment to the child and his family.

ASSESSING NEEDS FOR SUPPORT

When the child's medical condition has stabilized and the family can once again begin to think about recovery and discharge to home, the service coordinator or other member of the developmental team may begin to explore needs for support with the family. While direct discussion with the family is essential in establishing the areas in which they would see themselves needing additional support, a number of structured assessment measures are available to assess family function and need.

In the past, family assessment was usually designed to identify psychopathology. Some of the available assessment measures reflect this, such as measures of parental depression. The contemporary approach in providing emotional support to families of chronically ill children is to collaborate with the family so that they themselves may identify their own strengths as well as needs. Some of the family measures will assist in clarifying areas of strength and need.

Tools for family assessment

A number of needs surveys have been designed to evaluate service needs in families of children with disabilities; several have been developed specifically for families of children with special health care needs. (See Chapter 6.) These tend to focus on specific needs for information or a particular service.

Other measures are available that may assist in identifying particular needs for emotional support. One area that might be evaluated is that of overall family functioning. **The Family Environment Scale** (Moos and Moos, 1981) provides a parent-reported rating of areas such as family communication, cohesiveness and conflict. This may allow identification of strengths in family functioning. The **FACES III** (Olson et al., 1985) is a similar measure assessing family adaptability and cohesion.

The **Parenting Stress Index** (PSI) (Abidin, 1983) is a widely used measure designed to identify stress related to parenting a child with a disability. The PSI provides a cutoff point above which the family is felt to be demonstrating clinical levels of stress.

The **Impact-on-Family Scale** (Stein and Riessman, 1980) was designed to assess stress in mothers of chronically ill children. It assesses four dimensions of impact: financial, social/familial, personal strain, and mastery.

Coping Health Inventory for Parents (CHIP) (McCubbin et al., 1983) is a measure of coping patterns as families adapt to stresses in parenting a chronically ill child.

Stress in the sense of depression can be evaluated through a number of well-designed and validated depression indices. The **Beck Depression Inventory** (Beck et al., 1961) is a relatively brief questionnaire that could be a part of the family assessment measures packet.

Family support networks have become an area of increasing interest in understanding coping in the face of parenting a chronically ill child. Among the measures available to assess family support are:

- Carolina Parent Support Scale (Bristol, 1983)
- The Family Support Scale (Dunst, Trivette, and Deal, 1988)
- Questionnaire on Resources and Stress (Holroyd, 1987)

These measures look at the types and numbers of individuals identified by the family as providing them with different types of support (emotional, informational, etc.). The availability of support networks and the quality of the network (a few intimate supports vs. many less close) has been shown to represent an important stress mediator for families of chronically ill children (Kazak, 1989). Knowledge about whom the family view as supports may be helpful in problem solving around particular needs of the family.

Coping Strategies

Coping strategies for families as a unit and for individuals within the unit will vary greatly. Individuals may use coping techniques known as *defense mechanisms*. The common defenses defined by psychodynamic theory include *denial, displacement, intellectualization and projection*. If utilization of these defenses enables a parent to tolerate the tremendous emotional stress of their child's acute illness, then professionals must recognize this need. Some professionals become very concerned about the extent of denial that a parent may express in continuing to expect that their terminally ill child will recover. Most often the parent will recognize the reality of their child's condition even though denial may be his or her coping strategy. The problem comes when denial might result in the parent's not following through on a medical need.

In other instances, the parents' displacement of frustration in reaction to their powerlessness in dealing with their child's condition is directed at staff. Nursing staff and intervention staff need to be aware that parental antagonism may not be personally directed at staff members but reflects the pain experienced by the parents. Acknowledging the parents' pain, responding nondefensively, and being a good listener may help to reduce the parents' need to displace their frustration onto staff.

APPRECIATION FOR INDIVIDUAL CHARACTERISTICS OF FAMILIES

Although studies have attempted to identify shared characteristics of families of chronically ill children in terms of the types of stresses they experience, it is important to remember that, in fact, each family is unique. Ethnic, cultural, and religious influences will affect how members of a particular family cope with stress and relate to each other. These factors may also affect how the family deals with institutions and professionals. They also must certainly influence the parents' attitudes about their child's disability and possible death. Professionals working with the family need to be aware of how the family's ethnic background may potentially affect their coping with the child's illness. On the other hand, professionals need to be careful observers and sensitive questioners to understand the particular influences contributing to a family's response. Those professional disciplines with specific training in family assessment and interviewing, particularly social work and psychology, may be able to provide consultation to other team members in evaluating strategies to gather information on family needs and the various factors impacting on family functioning.

CHANGING NEEDS OF THE FAMILY OVER TIME

Given the fact that a chronically ill child typically will have repeated hospitalizations, it can be anticipated that family needs will change over time. A thorough exploration of family function and needs will probably be helpful at the time of initial identification of child and family. Subsequent hospitalization may require updating but not re-administration of the full assessment battery.

As parents become more familiar with their child's needs in relation to the medical condition and to available community resources for meeting those needs, previous needs for information and training may no longer be relevant. As time goes by, the parent will typically begin to have more questions about their child's developmental capability.

At *points of transition*, such as a move from early intervention program to a preschool program, the parent may once again be in need of information and assistance in accessing appropriate community resources.

Other transitions that are frequently stressful for the family are those having to do with *major shifts in the medical management plan*. When the physician determines that the child is stable enough for a reduction in home nursing service, the family may be relieved not to have another person in the home. For other families, however, there may be increased anxiety that the child's medical status will be jeopardized by the absence of the nurse. Similar ambivalent feelings may be engendered in the family in response to the planned removal of a tracheostomy. It is not uncommon for parents to question the wisdom of the physicians in the timing of these decisions. Families experiencing stress in relation to these issues should be encouraged to discuss them with the physicians and other relevant team members. The interventionist should be supportive of the family in helping them to initiate further dialogue. One must be cautious, however, not to get caught up in taking sides when parents disagree with physician decisions. While clarification about the reasons underlying decision-making can be requested, it is important for professionals and the family to arrive at a consensus as to the medical and development plan.

TRANSITION TO HOME CARE

Although this guide focuses on intervention during hospitalization, the intervention team plays an important role in assisting in transition to home care. Specific aspects of discharge planning are described in Chapter 6. This section will focus on typical areas of stress for families maintaining the chronically ill child at home.

Conflicts in the Medical Management Plan

The family will often continue to depend on hospital professionals to oversee the medical management plan at home in conjunction with the family pediatrician. Given the variety of medical specialists involved with a chronically ill child, it may occasionally happen that conflicting medical recommendations are provided by different physicians. Families are understandably distressed when this occurs, but they may not know how to resolve the conflict. It may also happen that one physician assumes the other is overseeing a medical problem, while in reality no one has assumed responsibility for that medical concern. It will be important, as time goes by, for families to recognize when these glitches in the medical management plan occur and to initiate a conference of the medical staff involved to resolve the problem. Initially however, it may require an intervention team member, most often the service coordinator, to support the family in seeking improved communication among the professionals involved. These issues may come up even when the child is an inpatient. When the child is at home, however, maintaining communication among the various specialists may be that much more difficult.

Utilizing Respite Care Services

The physical and emotional burden of caring for a chronically ill child at home is a serious one. Parents electing home management usually have a strong commitment to assuming personal responsibility for the care of their child. While not always the case, in many families it is the mother who assumes the majority of caregiving responsibility for the child. The father may be less familiar with caregiving needs, and in fact, not yet be comfortable when he has to provide for them. It is not unusual for this situation to result in family conflict. The mother may feel overburdened and believe that there is no one else capable of adequately caring for the child. The father may feel displaced in his role with the child and uncomfortable with his lack of competence in managing care. A family in this position may also not feel able to entrust the child to a respite care provider.

The interventionist may play an important role in helping the family to evaluate how the division of responsibility has been made and whether, in fact, this is an adaptive strategy for the family as a whole. In addition, the importance of utilizing respite might be explored with the family and information about respite resources discussed.

Coping with Home Nursing Care

The relationship with home nurses is a very sensitive one for families of chronically ill children. Often the family is dependent upon the security the nurse represents in providing for the medical needs of the child. And yet the family must adjust to the continuing presence of a non-family member in their midst.

The dependence on the availability of home nursing care may create stress for the family. Nursing agencies vary greatly in the consistency of skill level of the staff they provide. They may also vary in their reliability in hiring enough nurses to fill required shifts. It is not unusual for a family to learn at the last minute that the agency is unable to provide a nurse for a given shift or shifts. Negotiating with home nursing agencies is an important ability the family must develop, but they will usually require support from medical and intervention professionals to express their needs and concerns.

Other areas of conflict with home nursing have to do with issues of privacy and with cultural or attitudinal differences between the family and the nurse. One family described the stress they felt because they were uncomfortable discussing family issues or fighting with each other in front of the nurse. Another family felt that differences between themselves and the nurse in culturally-based attitudes about child-rearing, and even food, put a strain on the relationship. When these issues cannot be resolved even after open discussion, it may be better for the family to request a change in the nurse assigned.

In other situations the nurse may develop a very close relationship with the family, such that he or she is viewed almost as a family member. This may be potentially stressful for the nurse if she becomes enmeshed in preexisting family conflicts.

Ongoing support from the intervention team may be important to some families if they are to be effective employers of in-home service providers and effective advocates for their child with special health care needs.

BEREAVEMENT

SUPPORT TO FAMILIES

The death of a child is devastating, traumatic, and painful for parents. It "represents the loss of future dreams, relationships, experiences and fantasies that have not yet been enjoyed" (Knapp, 1987). Although the parents of a chronically ill child have already had to grieve the loss of the "perfect child," this does not lessen the impact of the child's death upon the parents.

Helping parents cope should begin at a point prior to the child's actual death in situations where the terminal stage of the child's illness is recognized. Even when death is anticipated, parents may respond with shock in much the same way as when death is sudden. A bereavement plan instituted within the PICU structure will be helpful for both families and staff. This program should provide step-by-step procedures for staff to follow in conjunction with the death of the child on the unit. These procedures may relate to such issues as removal of tubes and equipment, allowing families to bathe and dress the child's body, and assisting in identifying resources for the funeral or burial (Antonacci, 1988; Moseley et al., 1988).

While each family and family member will respond in some unique way to the death, there are some typical patterns seen in many families. Parents tend to describe their initial response as one of disbelief and numbness, even if the death was long expected. Typically, after about two to three weeks, the numbness gives way to a lengthy period of mourning. Generally, the manner in which parents mourn or respond to the death of a child varies, but Knapp (1987) has identified six similarities:

- Fear that the memories they have of their child will fade away
- An eventual need to talk about their tragic experience and the memories of their child
- A need to search for some cause or rational reason for the loss
- A change in values, especially for parents who struggled through a long terminal illness with a child
- Shadow grief such that no amount of time will ever totally resolve the grief

There is nothing anyone can do to alleviate the pain of losing a child. But there are a number of things that interventionists can do to provide support to grieving parents; they include:

- Be available to both parents; fathers need support as well as mothers, and each parent may express feelings in different ways.
- Don't avoid families or expect them to call you; call them.
- Listen to feelings, remember there is little you can say, but often parents have few people who are willing to listen to them.
- Use simple touch; often touch means more than talk.
- Make facilitative statements. (See Table 13.) Understand that parents do not need to hear rationalizations about their child's death.
- Help build memories. Make a "Book of Memories" for the family, including photos of the child with written memories the various staff members have of the child. Provide tangible memories, such as a drawing the child made, a hospital identification band, a lock of hair, or a favorite toy the child had. Should the family indicate that they don't want these mementos, keep them for several months because families often change their minds about this later.
- Be aware of ritual practices of the family's ethnic or religious background.
- Offer to participate in the funeral or memorial service if appropriate.
- Attend funeral/memorial service.
- Remember important dates (child's birthday, anniversary of death, Christmas) with cards, phone calls, or visits.
- Refer family to local resources (bereavement groups, counselors, clergy, etc.)
- Remember that it takes years for parents to adjust to the loss of a child, and that grief is never totally resolved.

One parent in Knapp's (1987) study summarized her feelings: "My son died 13

Table 13
Facilitative Statements to Say to Bereaved Families

Say:	Instead of:
"I'm so sorry."	"I know how you feel."
"I imagine it hurts a lot to see Johnny so close to death."	"It was for the best."
"I'm here to listen." "I'm going to miss Sally, too."	"She would have suffered if she had lived."
"I'm going to miss Stevie's wonderful smile."	"Your child would have been a burden to you as he was."
Use child's name.	"At least you have your (spouse, other children, health)."
	"You're young, you can have another."

years ago...Although I don't cry anymore as often as I used to, my life is not the same...It will never be the same...nor do I expect it to be."

SUPPORT FOR SIBLINGS

Just as living with a chronically ill child impacts upon siblings, the death of that child has a significant impact as well. Siblings are often overlooked in the grieving family, especially if they are not openly expressing their grief in a destructive manner (acting out, skipping school, etc.). Naturally, children of different ages will express their grief in different ways, but all will have some emotional response. According to the nationwide support group, "Compassionate Friends" (1987), children may experience the loss of a sibling in one or more of the following ways:

- Sleep disturbances
- Restlessness or fatigue
- Anger toward themselves, other people, God, or the sibling who has died
- Fear of their safety and the safety of others in their family
- Feeling of rejection from parents who are distracted, irritable, or inattentive
- Trouble paying attention and remembering;
- Mood swings between feeling very good and very bad
- Guilt about what they did or did not do for their brother or sister, for enjoying themselves, and even for just surviving

Interventionists can play a particularly helpful role by providing some support to the siblings during the grieving process, especially when the parents are still in a period of shock and intense mourning. Interventionists can provide support simply by listening and encouraging them to verbalize their feelings. Interventionists can also remind children that their feelings are normal and that they should not be ashamed of them. In addition, interventionists should remind children that it is appropriate:

- To cry and feel depressed
- To want to copy some of their brother or sister's habits and interests
- To live "in the past" for a period of time
- To have fun and enjoy life, to laugh again
- To forgive themselves for the fights, arguments, and/or bad thoughts they had about their brother or sister
- To go on living.

(Compassionate Friends, 1987)

Often children try to protect their parents by not revealing their despair. Interventionists can help the parent communicate with the child by pointing out typical behavior of grieving siblings.

SUPPORT TO PROFESSIONAL STAFF

Unfortunately, most interventionists working with chronically ill children will themselves need to deal with the pain surrounding the loss of a child under their care. This pain may be exacerbated if the interventionist has not previously experienced this kind of loss or has not received training in dealing with grief. The intensity of such grief may be affected by the following factors:

- Prior experiences with grief and loss

- Amount of involvement with the family
- Additional professional and personal stresses placed upon the interventionist

Regardless of its intensity, professional staff will need to work through their grief in order to continue to be effective in this work. Staff members can help themselves and each other in the following ways:

- Giving themselves permission to grieve
- Utilizing peer supports to talk about feelings and/or memories of the child
- Recognizing their own limits during the initial grieving period
- Attending and/or participating in the funeral or memorial service
- Pulling together photos of the child to make a "memory book" for the grieving family
- Scheduling time to visit with the grieving family
- Expressing feelings in a journal
- Reducing stress through exercise, relaxation techniques and/or medication

Many of these suggestions are similar to methods that are effective in helping the grieving family, but they are of equal benefit to the professional staff. Though the grief that a staff person feels could not equal that of the family, she too has suffered a loss. This loss needs to be acknowledged. Building her own memories and reflecting upon her work with the child will not only help the interventionist cope with the present crisis, but will add to her professional growth in supporting families with chronically ill children in the future.

REFERENCES

Abidin, R. (1983). *The Parenting Stress Index.* Charlottesville, VA: Pediatric Psychology Press.

Antonacci, M. (1988). Sudden death: Helping bereaved parents in the PICU. *Critical Care Nurse,* 10, 65-70.

Bailey, D., Simeonsson, R., Winton, P., Huntington, G., Comfort, M., Isbell, P., O'Donnell, K., & Helm, J. (1986). Family focused intervention: A functional model for planning, implementing and evaluating family services in early intervention. *Journal of the Division of Early Childhood* 10(2), 156-171.

Beck, A., Ward, C., Mendelson, M., Mock, J. & Erbaugh, J. (1961). Beck depression inventory: An inventory for measuring depression. *Archives of General Psychiatry*, 4, 53-63.

Bennett, F.C. (1987). The effectiveness of early intervention for infants at increased biological risk. In M. Guralnick and F. Bennett, *The Effectiveness of Early Intervention for At Risk and Handicapped Children,* (pp. 79-114). Orlando, FL: Academic Press.

Bristol, M. (1983). *Carolina Parent Support Scale.* Chapel Hill, NC: Frank Porter Graham Child Development Center.

Bryant, D. & Ramey, C. (1987). An analysis of the effectiveness of early intervention programs for environmentally at risk children. In M. Guralnick and F. Bennett, *The Effectiveness of Early Intervention for At Risk and Handicapped Children,* (pp. 33-78). Orlando, FL: Academic Press.

The Compassionate Friends, Inc. (1987). *When a brother or sister dies*. Oak Brook, IL: The Compassionate Friends, Inc.

Dunst, C., Trivette, C. & Deal, A. (1988) *Enabling and empowering families: Principles and guidelines for practice*. Cambridge, MA: Brookline Books.

Holroyd, J. (1987). Questionnaire on Resources and Stress. VT: Brandon Clinical Psychology Publishing Co., Inc.

Kazak, A. (1989). Families of chronically ill children: A systems and social ecological model of adaptation and challenge. *Journal of Consulting and Clinical Psychology*, 57, 25-30.

Knapp, R.J. (1987). When a child dies: How parents react to and cope with one of life's most devastating losses. *Psychology Today*, 21, 60-67.

McCubbin, H., McCubbin, M., Patterson, J., Cauble, A., Wilson, L., & Warwick, W. (1983). CHIP - Coping health inventory for parents: An assessment of parental coping patterns in the care of the chronically ill child. *Journal of Marriage and the Family*, 45(2), 359-370.

Moos, R. & Moos, B. (1981). *Family Environment Scale: Manual*. Palo Alto, CA: Consulting Psychologist Press.

Moseley, J., Logan, S., Tolle, S., & Bentley, J. (1988). Developing a Bereavement Program in a University Hospital Setting. *Oncology Nursing Fundamentals*, 15, 151-155.

Olson, D., Portner, J., Lavee, Y. (1985). *FACES III*. St. Paul, MN: Family Social Science. University of Minnestoa.

Stein, R. & Riessman, C. (1980). The Development of an Impact on Family Scale: Preliminary findings. *Medical Care,* 18, 465-472.

Chapter 8

The Future for Children with Chronic Illness

Kathy S. Katz, Ph.D.

We may anticipate in the coming years that medical advances will continue to expand the numbers and longevity of children with chronic illness. We have seen the enormous increase in survival rates of children from the NICU. While research suggests that incidence of severe degrees of complications, such as bronchopulmonary dysplasia and intraventricular hemorrhage, has been somewhat reduced, the actual number of children discharged with some degree of special care needs has increased (Hack et al., 1991).

We have seen that medical technology can enhance survival but can itself produce chronic conditions that require ongoing management. Hospital stays are prolonged for these children, and rehospitalizations occur frequently. The majority of children currently surviving with chronic health conditions a decade ago would have remained hospitalized in acute or chronic care facilities for months or even years. Today many of these children are entering the community. They are able to remain with their families, thanks to a complex network of community supports. The variety of support services required by the chronically ill infant and his family can only be successfully provided through the collaborative efforts of multiple community agencies. Much work remains to be done in expanding and enhancing the effectiveness of inter-agency coordination and in the availability of community services designed for chronically ill children. This section will focus on current models for exemplary services for children with special health care needs and additional future service needs.

MODELS FOR INTER-AGENCY COLLABORATION

To provide better coordination of services to children with special health care needs, a number of model service programs have been developed. One model that has been piloted in Iowa (Nelson, 1987) is a regional center at which professionals from health, social services, and educational agencies provide collaborative services for children with chronic health problems. At these centers the children receive special evaluations and coordination of services to deal with health-related educational and behavioral problems.

A model of this type reduces the need for parents to deal with a variety of agencies and professionals at different sites. This reduces the cumbersome logistical problems of transporting a child with technologic equipment to multiple service providers. It also enhances the opportunity to maintain close communication among professionals working with the family.

Another successful support model for technology-dependent children has been that of a coordinating center to assist in the transition of the child from the hospital to the home setting. These programs have been established under state aegis to help in the coordination of the Medicare waiver services for home-based care for technology-dependent children.

The coordinating centers provide a case management role in arranging the various equipment and home nursing services that will be required by the family. The time required to get these services in place is enormous and would be overwhelming for a family about to assume care of the infant at home. The coordinating centers take responsibility for organizing the financial arrangements for home care and for assisting in resolving conflict among the family and any of the vendors providing services.

Additional models are needed in many geographic areas, particularly rural ones, that will provide enhanced inter-agency collaboration in services for chronically ill children. This will help to lessen the additional burden placed on parents needing to arrange services for their child.

NEED FOR PRIMARY MEDICAL CARE

For a very prolonged period the family of the chronically ill child must rely on medical specialists, usually affiliated with tertiary care centers, to manage their child's medical care. This remains true for a period of time even after discharge. It is not unusual for the families to drive several hundred miles weekly, keeping appointments with the various medical specialists. In the early weeks following discharge, families may return to the tertiary center for consultation even for common childhood illnesses that their child might contract. As the child's condition becomes more stable, however, it is preferable for the family to seek regular medical care from a **primary physician**.

The primary care physician is the medical professional who assumes responsibility for providing the child with regular immunizations, monitoring growth, and assuming medical management of common childhood ailments. Primary care physicians are usually prepared in training programs in family medicine (formerly general practice) or pediatrics. Training of primary care physicians focuses heavily on preventive care. A difficulty arises in that even those primary care physicians with pediatric training may have had limited exposure to children with chronic health care needs. A number of primary care physicians may not feel comfortable managing the regular pediatric care of a child with complex health needs. Others may be able to address the primary medical needs but not be able to provide adequate support to families around nutrition and growth issues or early intervention needs.

This is a situation in which technology has proceeded more rapidly than training opportunities have been able to address. For many primary physicians currently in practice, it would have been totally unexpected that infants with such complex medical needs could be managed at home, as these children have been, in the past few years. During their training, few of these physicians would have had exposure to children with chronic conditions other than in acute inpatient care.

In order for children with special health care needs and their families to be adequately served in the community, more primary physicians familiar with general health needs of these children must be prepared. Several physician-training programs are currently attempting this, such as that at Michigan State University (Desguin, 1986). These physician-training models provide exposure to the varied needs of chronically ill children to participants in pediatric residency programs . The programs include didactic training in normal and abnormal development with an emphasis on developmental implications of special health care needs. Residents participate in outpatient primary health care of children with chronic conditions. A unique feature is the usual requirement that the resident spend time in the home of a chronically ill child to become familiar with what caregiving entails on a day-to-day basis for these families.

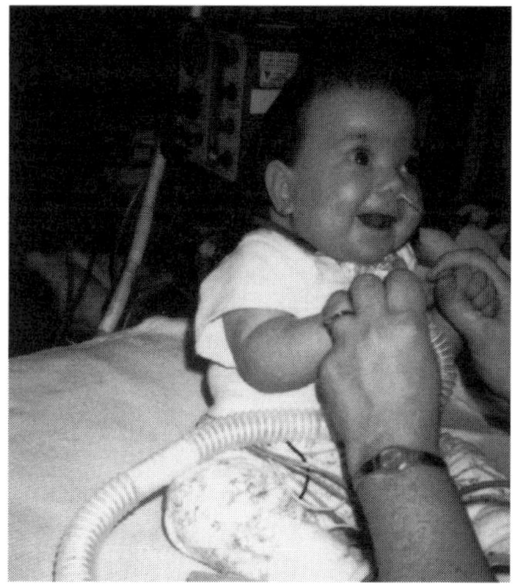

Family-centered care for children with special health care needs has been widely publicized, especially through the efforts of the former Surgeon General C. Everett Koop. The impact of this philosophy has been widely disseminated in nursing training and is beginning to expand into physician training, as well. It is hoped in the coming years that training in primary care needs of chronically ill children will become an integral part of the preparation of family physicians and pediatricians. This will greatly enhance the support to families of chronically ill children in the community. Early intervention personnel in university training hospitals may perhaps be able to bring these training needs to the awareness of the individuals within their institutions who are responsible for developing medical and nursing training curricula.

TRAINING NEEDS FOR EARLY INTERVENTION PERSONNEL

In the same way that primary care physicians may have limited exposure to children with chronic illness, the majority of early intervention professionals have also had limited experience with these children. Training of allied health professionals, such as physical or occupational therapists, usually includes experience with individuals with health conditions, but rarely in the past has it been with young children with chronic health care needs. For the most part, this has also been true of speech pathologists and psychologists, and it has been especially true of early childhood educators. Educators, until only the last few years, were prepared specifically to provide services to children in classrooms. Children would only be accepted into classrooms if their health was stable. With more health-impaired children living at home and with an expanded mandate for states to provide for their educational needs, early interventionists must now frequently provide services to children with complex health problems. This may occur through home-based services or in center-based classrooms.

Increasingly, training programs for early interventionists are including didactic, and sometimes applied, experience with chronically ill infants. For several years, the Georgetown University Child Development Center has had an Interdisciplinary Training Program for early intervention professionals with an emphasis on service provision to medically fragile infants. The participating individuals are provided didactic and direct service experiences with inpatient children, in high risk follow-up clinics, in home-based intervention and in center-based classrooms serving children with special health care needs. In this way, these young professionals are sensitized to the needs of the family as a whole, as well as to the particular implication of the health condition.

In the coming years, more in-service training opportunities should be available for early intervention and social service personnel to prepare them for meeting the special needs of chronically ill children and their families.

NEEDS FOR RESPITE CARE

Availability of respite care for families caring for chronically ill children at home is essential if these families are to tolerate the continuing stress of managing the children at home. Additionally, in order for parents to be able to return to work, day-care providers prepared to handle the child's health care needs must be available. This is one area in which most communities are severely lacking in available resources. It is an area that many families cite as a major needed support (Delaney and Zolondick, 1991).

One approach is to prepare home daycare providers to perform such procedures as CPR, suctioning, and gavage feeding, so that they may provide respite in the child's home or their own. One such program, through the New York State Department of Health, has focused on developing and implementing a network of medically-skilled respite care providers (Sherman, 1988). Other programs, such as the Prescribed Pediatric Extended Care project in Florida (Pierce and Freedman, 1987), offer day medical care to medically or technology-dependent children in a group day-care setting. Expansion of programs of this type in other regions is very much needed.

FINANCING OF COMMUNITY-BASED CARE FOR CHILDREN WITH SPECIAL HEALTH CARE NEEDS

Another area frequently cited by parents as a major contributor to the stresses of caring for their chronically ill child at home is the financing of that care. Increased availability of financing resources, such as Medicaid waivers, has greatly enhanced the feasibility of supporting a chronically ill child at home. However, the complexity of orchestrating a variety of financing measures is an overwhelming task for most families.

The availability of individuals or collaborating agencies that will guide families through the maze of potential financing resources would be a an invaluable support to families. Programs such as the Coordinating Center for Home and Community Care of Maryland (Force and Kaufman, 1988) have assisted families in securing medical services necessary for their technology-dependent child at home and coordinated the funding sources. They have also been able to demonstrate the cost effectiveness of home- based care as compared with hospital care, thus convincing third party payers as to the wisdom of supporting home-based care . Greater inter-agency coordination is needed, however, as well as policy initiatives for third party payers to increase the likelihood of support of community-based care.

NEEDS FOR PARENT-TO-PARENT SUPPORT

An additional avenue for support sometimes overlooked by professionals is that of parent-to-parent support for families of chronically ill children. These contacts provide important emotional support for families. They also provide an avenue for group advocacy efforts that will continue to be a means for parents to make an impact on policy development for chronically ill children.

For these groups to be maintained, they must have a stable source of funding. It has been suggested that this might come from federal or state revenues. Additionally, individuals in these groups may need formal training in effective advocacy techniques and ways to influence policy. Programs such as the Federation for Children with Special Needs are designed to increase parent involvement in the health care of their children. This program also promotes the linkage of parents and health professionals to improve communication and collaboration between these groups. It is felt that the greatest impact on policy will probably be effected through this type of collaboration.

In summary, a number of needs of families of chronically ill children must be addressed in the coming years if there is to be continued expansion of community-based care. These include

- Increased collaboration of medical, developmental, social service, educational, and financing agencies in coordinating home-based services
- Availability of primary care providers familiar with needs of chronically ill children
- Early intervention and allied health professionals comfortable with service delivery to medically fragile young children
- Needs for respite care resources prepared to deal with children with special health care needs
- Increased financing resources for community-based care
- Availability of parent-to-parent support groups

Early intervention professionals working with families of chronically ill children may help these families by identifying resources in their community that would provide for these needs. The next step will be to identify the gaps in service in the local community. Early interventionists and families must then work collaboratively to advocate for the services not available in the community that represent necessary supports for families. It is only through these collaborative efforts that the needs of chronically ill children and their families can truly be served.

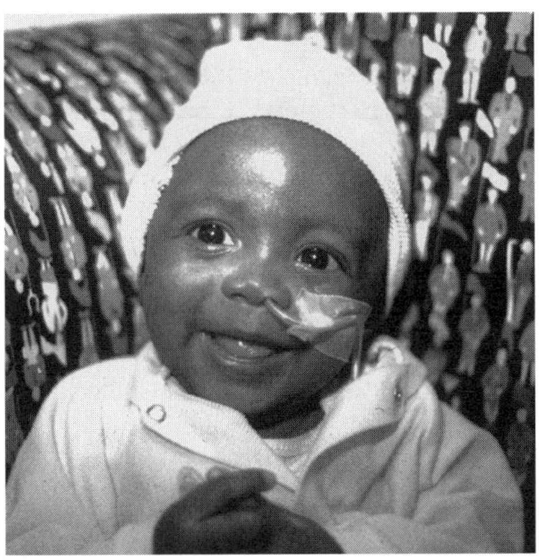

REFERENCES

Delaney, N. and Zolondick, K. (1991). Daycare for technology-dependent infants and children: A new alternative. *Journal of Perinatal and Neonatal Nursing,* 5, 80-85.

Desguin, B. (1986). Chronic Illness in Children. *American Journal of Diseases in Children,* 140, 1246-1249.

Force, J. & Kaufman, J. (1988, September). *A Model for Home and Community Care for the Technology Assisted.* Poster presented at the U.S. Surgeon General's Conference Campaign '88: Building Community-based Service Systems for Children with Special Health Care Needs (Washington, DC).

Hack, M., Hobar, J., Mallory, M., Tyson, J., Wright, E., & Wright, L. (1991). Very low birthweight outcomes of the National Institute of Child Health and Human Development Neonatal Network. *Pediatrics,* 87: 587-599.

Nelson, R. (1987, June). *Iowa Program for Children with Special Health Care Needs.* Poster presented at the Surgeon General's Conference: Campaign '87 Commitment to Family Centered Coordinated Care for Children with Special Health Care Needs. (Houston, TX).

Pierce, P. & Freedman, S. (1987, June). *Prescribed pediatric extended care.* Poster presented at the Surgeon General's Conference: Campaign '87 Commitment to Family Centered Coordinated Care for Children with Special Health Care Needs. (Houston, TX).

Sherman, B. (1988). Home-based family support services for chronically ill children and their families. In Bureau of Maternal and Child Health, Putting great ideas into action: *On behalf of children with special health care needs and their families.* Second Annual National SPRANS Workshop Proceedings. Washington, DC: U.S. Department of Health and Human Services, 71.

Appendix A

HEARING ASSESSMENT INSTRUMENTS

Auditory Brainstem Response (ABR)
Type of Measure: Test of the Integrity of the Auditory Mechanism
Age Range: Birth-Adulthood
Administration Requisites: Evoked response equipment, electrodes, earphones, sedation for ages 6 months - 8 years
Administration Time: 60 minutes

Behavioral Audiometry (Behavioral Observation Audiometry, Visual Reinforcement Audiometry, conditioned play and conventional techniques)
Type of Measure: Test of hearing perception
Age Range: Birth-Adulthood
Administration Requisites: Audiometer
Administration Time: 30 - 60 minutes

Tympanometry
Type of Measure: Test of Eustachian Tube and middle ear function
Age Range: Birth-Adulthood
Administration Requisites: Tympanometer
Administration Time: Less than 5 minutes

LANGUAGE ASSESSMENT INSTRUMENTS

Bzoch, K.R. & League, R. (1991). Receptive-Expressive Emergent Language Scale (REEL-2) Austin, TX: Pro-Ed
Type of Measure: Normed referenced in-depth test
Age Range: Birth to 36 months
Content Areas: Receptive Language, Expressive Language
Administration Time: 15 - 30 minutes

Coplan, J. (1984). The Early Language Milestone Scale (ELM Scale) Tulsa, OK: Modern Education Corp.
Type of Measure: Norm referenced screening test
Age Range: Birth to 3 years
Content Areas: Auditory Expression, Auditory Reception, Visual
Administration Time: 5 -10 minutes

Furuno, S., Inatsuka, T.T., O'Reilly, K.A., Hosaka, C.M., Zeisloft-Falbey, B., &. Allman, T. (1988). Hawaii Early Learning Profile (HELP)Palo Alto, CA: VORT Corp.
Type of Measure: Criterion-referenced in-depth test
Age Range: Birth to 3 years

Content Areas: Cognitive, fine motor, gross motor, expressive language, socio-emotional and self-help
Administration time: 15 - 60 minutes

Rossetti, Louis. (1990). The Rossetti Infant-Toddler Language Scale
East Moline, IL: LinguiSystems, Inc.
Type of Measure: Norm-referenced in-depth test
Age Range: Birth to 3 years
Content Areas: Interaction-Attachment, Pragmatics, Gesture,Play, Language Comprehension, Language Expression
Administration Time: 30 - 60 minutes

ORAL-MOTOR/FEEDING REFERENCES

Blager, F. & Hynes, P. (1982). Speech and Language Assessment and Treatment of Handicapped Infants and Preschool Children. Denver, CO: University of Colorado.

Jelm, Judy. (1990). Oral-Motor/Feeding Rating Scale. Tucson, AZ: Therapy Skill Builders.

Morris, S.E. and M.D. Klein. (1987). Pre-Feeding Skills. Tucson, AZ: Therapy Skill Builders.

Appendix B

Feeding Equipment

- Preemie Nipples are easier to suck. They are made of soft material, have a small crosscut opening and facilitate infants with low energy levels and weak sucks.

- Specialized nipples for cleft palate infants are designed to assist infants who have difficulty building up the negative pressure needed for sucking. They are frequently longer and may be thinner than other nipples.

- Specialized bottles are also used. Some help regulate liquid flow and others are designed to allow children to be positioned in prone or side-lying while drinking.

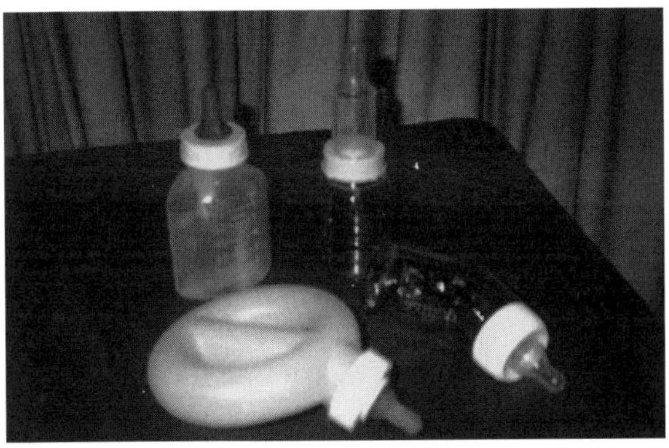

- Lidded cups with slits instead of spouts are used to assist children in learning cup-drinking oral-motor postures.

- Spoons that are relatively flat, do not break when bitten, fit the child's mouth, are easy for the feeder to hold and are coated to minimize temperature or taste changes are preferred.

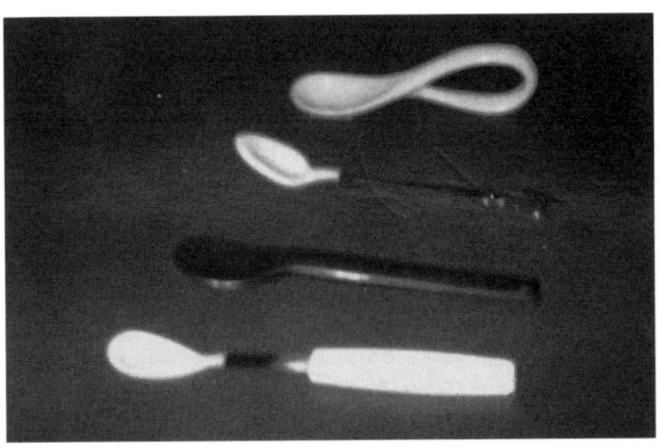

Appendix C

Survey for Families of Children with Special Health Care Needs

Child's Name ______________________ Your Relationship to Child ______________

Listed below are some of the concerns expressed by parents of children with health care needs with which they would like help. Please read each statement.

If it is not a need for you at this time, circle number 1.

If you are not sure about whether you need or would like help in this area, circle number 2.

If it is a need for you and you would like help at this time, please circle number 3.

This information will be confidential to the developmental team.

	I do not need help with this	Not sure	I need help with this
A. Needs for Information			
1. I need more information about my child's health condition or development.	**1**	**2**	**3**
2. I need more information on the services that are available for my child.	**1**	**2**	**3**
3. I need more information about services that my child might need in the future.	**1**	**2**	**3**
4. I want information about how my child will function in the future.	**1**	**2**	**3**
5. I need more information about/or applications for public programs, i.e., WIC, SSI, Housing.	**1**	**2**	**3**
6. I need more information about how children grow and develop.	**1**	**2**	**3**
7. I need more information about how to teach, play, or talk with my child.	**1**	**2**	**3**
8. I need more information about how to manage my child's sleep patterns.	**1**	**2**	**3**
9. I need more information on managing my child's feeding.	**1**	**2**	**3**
10. I need more information about how to handle my child's or his/her sibling's behavior.	**1**	**2**	**3**

Adapted with permission from:

Bailey, D.,& Simeonsson, R. (1985). *Family Needs Survey.* Chapel Hill: Frank Porter Graham Child Development Ctr.

Kaufman, J. & Lichtenstein, K.A. *The Family as Care Manager: Home Care Coordination for Medically Fragile Children.* Washington, DC: Georgetown University Child Development Center.

Developed by: Kathy S. Katz , PhD and Cindy Baker, MA

Washington, DC: Georgetown University Child Development Center. 1989

	I do not need help with this	Not sure	I need help with this
B. Needs for Support			
1. I need to have more time for myself.	1	2	3
2. I would like an opportunity to talk with another family of a special needs child.	1	2	3
3. I would like information about a parent support group.	1	2	3
4. I need reading material about other parents who have a child similar to mine.	1	2	3
5. I would like to be able to discuss problems with a friend.	1	2	3
6. I would like to have a referral to talk to a counselor (psychologist, social worker or psychiatrist).			
7. I would like to talk to a minister or other religious counselor.	1	2	3
8. I would like more time to talk with my child's service coordinator or other developmental team members.			
C. Explaining to Others			
1 I need more help in how to explain my child's condition to family members, significant other/spouse, child's siblings, friends, others.	1	2	3
2. My significant other/spouse needs help understanding and accepting my child's condition.	1	2	3
D. Family Issues			
1. Our family needs help in learning to resolve conflicts.	1	2	3
2. Our family needs help in learning how to support each other in stressful times	1	2	3
3. Our family needs help in deciding who will be responsible for which household or child care tasks	1	2	3
E. Needs for My Home			
1. I need safety equipment in my home, (e. g. , smoke detector, fire extinguisher.)	1	2	3
2. My utilities/appliances need updating for my child's safety (e. g. , electrical, water heater, heating system)	1	2	3
3. I need special adaptive equipment such as stroller, pronestander, for my child.	1	2	3
4. I need a telephone.	1	2	3
5. I need to make changes in my home environment that have not been mentioned.	1	2	3
6. I need specific guidelines to handle problems that arise with equipment vendors (e.g., medical supplies) or nursing agencies.	1	2	3
7. I need to know who to call in case of an emergency.	1	2	3

	I do not need help with this	Not sure	I need help with this
8. I need a plan for my other children in case I need to leave quickly.	1	2	3
9. I need a plan for my child with health care needs in case I need to leave quickly.	1	2	3
10. I need a source for formula.	1	2	3
11. I need regular infant equipment or supplies (crib, carseat).	1	2	3
12. I need assistance in locating/ordering baby supplies.	1	2	3
13. I need assistance with transportation.	1	2	3
F. Needs for Medical Care, Therapy, and Community Services			
1. I need help locating a clinic or pediatrician who understands my child's special needs.	1	2	3
2. I need specific guidelines for when to call my pediatrician.	1	2	3
3. I need specific guidelines for when to go to the emergency room or to readmit my child to the hospital.	1	2	3
4. I need help locating a pharmacist or other medical supplier.	1	2	3
5. I need home nursing to help care for my child.	1	2	3
6. I need guidelines for dealing with specific problems with my home nurses.	1	2	3
7. I need additional training in caring for my child's health needs.	1	2	3
8. I need to be trained in CPR (cardiopulmonary resuscitation).	1	2	3
9. I need alternate caregivers to be trained in CPR.	1	2	3
10. I need help locating babysitters or respite care providers who are willing and able to care for my child.	1	2	3
11. I need a plan for child care in case of my own illness.	1	2	3
12. I need assistance in locating child care or preschool for my other children.	1	2	3
13. I need help in locating therapists for my child (OT, PT, Speech, etc.).	1	2	3
14. I need help in coordinating medical or developmental recommendations.	1	2	3
G. Financial Needs			
1. I need more help in paying for expenses such as food, housing, medical care, clothing, transportation, therapy, babysitting, day care and other services.	1	2	3
2. I need more help paying for toys that my child needs.	1	2	3

3. I need more help in getting special equipment for my child's needs.	**1**	**2**	**3**
4 I or my signifant other /spouse need more counseling or help in getting a job.	**1**	**2**	**3**

Needs that I'm concerned about which have not been mentioned:

____

____

____

____

____

____

____

Thank you for your time. Your service coordinator will be discussing your responses with you.

Appendix D

PROJECT HEADED HOME

Managing My Child's Medical Needs

Name: ______________________________

Please answer the following questions to let us know how comfortable you feel in terms of these technical management areas.

Circle #1 if you feel comfortable doing the task independently.
Circle #2 if you do the task with guidance.
Circle #3 if you are not comfortable doing the task yourself.
Circle #4 not applicable (N/A) if the question does not apply to your child.

	Comfortable Doing Independently	With Guidance	Not Comfortable Doing	N/A
1. I can tell when my child is ill.	1	2	3	4
2. I know what to do for my child when he/she is sick.	1	2	3	4
3. I know my child's medications.	1	2	3	4
4. I know how to administer my child's medications.	1	2	3	4
5. I know when my child is having trouble breathing.	1	2	3	4
6. I know how to do breathing treatments.	1	2	3	4
7. I know when, why, and how to use the nebulizer.	1	2	3	4
8. I know how to manage my child's apnea monitor.	1	2	3	4
9. I know how to do CPR.	1	2	3	4
10. I feel comfortable holding my child when he/she has tubes and monitors attached.	1	2	3	4
11. I feel I can explain my child's medical problems to family and friends.	1	2	3	4
12. I feel comfortable bathing and dressing my child.	1	2	3	4
13. I feel comfortable feeding my child.	1	2	3	4
14. I feel comfortable taking my child outside the house.	1	2	3	4

Managing My Child's Medical Needs (continued)

Name: ______________________________________

	Comfortable Doing Independently	With Guidance	Not Comfortable Doing	N/A
15. I feel comfortable moving my child to different areas to play.	1	2	3	4
16. I can suction my child when he/she has excess secretions.	1	2	3	4
17. I can care for my child's tracheostomy.	1	2	3	4
18. I can do tube feeding.	1	2	3	4
19. I know how to manage my child's oxygen equipment.	1	2	3	4
20. I feel comfortable taking my child out of the house with monitors and/or oxygen.	1	2	3	4

Appendix E

INDIVIDUALIZED FAMILY SERVICE PLAN

Child's name: David Q Date: February 15, 19—
DOB: 2/6/19—
CA: 12 months, 9 days

BACKGROUND HISTORY
Family members:
David Q, Susan Q (mother), and Mrs. P (grandmother)

Summary to date:
David Q is a one year old little boy who was born at 34 weeks gestation. He was in the NICU and then PICU at Georgetown Hospital for almost six months because of ventilator dependency. He was on the ventilator for most of that period and he had both a tracheostomy and a gastrostomy tube placed. He has a severe neuromuscular disorder which is currently undiagnosed, but effects his overall muscle tone, including respiration and oral feeding.

David lives at home with his mother and grandmother. He is followed by an HMO for medical care and receives developmental services through the Visiting Nurses Association. David has been rehospitalized on the PICU three times over the past several months for respiratory infections.

Measures Administered	Date Given	Chronological Age	Score
Bayley Mental	1/25/—	11 months, 19 days	<50 - 7.6 month age equivalent
Bayley Motor	1/25/—	11 months, 19 days	<50 - 5.3 month age equivalent
Neurological	1/25/—	11 months, 19 days	Abnormal secondary to severe hypotonia and muscle weakness
Audiological Evaluation	1/25/—	11 months, 19 days	Failed (follow-up with ENT scheduled)
Receptive-Expressive Emergent Language Scale (REEL)	1/25/—	11 months, 19 days	Receptive: 9-10 month equivalent Expressive: not scoreable

IFSP Sample (continued)

Child and Family Strengths:

Child's Strengths:

1. David is very alert and aware of what's going on in his environment.
2. David has age appropriate understanding of language.
3. David can now sit independently.
4. David has improved head control.
5. David can reach and grasp objects easily.
6. David does lots of oral-motor exploration with his hands and with toys.
7. David has a good established routine at home.

Family's Strengths:

1. Mother can handle all of David's medical needs.
2. Mother has extensive knowledge of David's various medical and developmental needs.
3. Mother is aware of many community resources and has been able to access a number of these.
4. Mother receives some respite time away from David when her mother takes care of David.
5. Mother is aware of David's developmental abilities and has maximized them.
6. Mother is very invested in all aspects of David and his care.

IFSP Sample (continued)

PROPOSED PLAN

Functional Outcomes/ Needs	Strategies	Person Responsible/ Timeline
1. Ms. Q would like to receive support from other parents of developmentally disabled children through a parent support group.	a. Identify local parent support group options.	Service coordinator inquire by 3/10
	b. Choose and attend an appropriate parent group.	Ms. Q by 4/7
2. Ms. Q will have increased personal time.	a. Identify possible respite care options for David.	Service coordinator by 3/31
	b. Attempt to recruit baby sitters through local nursing school programs.	Service coordinator by 3/31
3. David will have the opportunity to engage in socialization and play with other infants/toddlers.	a. Determine David's susceptibility to infection from pediatrician.	Ms. Q by 4/15
	b. Identify appropriate local play group options, if any.	Service coordinator by 3/17
	c. Attempt to secure infant development program services in a classroom-based setting.	Ms. Q through local Child Find program - - ongoing
4. David will be able to begin feeding by mouth.	a. Increase oral-motor exploration of objects and tolerance of textures through speech and language intervention and occupational therapy	VNA OT, and SLP - - on going
	b. Hospital team speech pathologist to coordinate with VNA speech therapist re: pre-feeding goals for David.	Home therapist to contact hospital team speech pathologist by 4/15.
	c. Ms. Q will receive suggestions for oral-motor activities for David.	VNA OT, and SLP

IFSP Sample (continued)

Functional Outcomes/ Needs	Strategies	Person Responsible/ Timeline
5. David will increase his ability to communicate his needs through the use of sign language.	a. Home based speech therapist will increase the number of signs David is exposed to in individual therapy.	Hospital SLP and VNA therapist- -ongoing
	b. Ms. Q will be provided a list and demonstration of signs to include in her interaction with David.	VNA SLP therapist by 4/15
6. David's hearing status will be clarified.	Results of ENT evaluation and repeat audiological testing.	Ms. Q and audiologist
7. David will be able to pull up to stand against furniture.	Continue PT and OT services through VNA.	Ms. Q and VNA - - ongoing

Responsible People:

Susan Q, David's mother

Cindy, MA
Infant Specialist
Service Coordinator

Sharon, MA, SLP-CCC
Speech-Language Pathologist

Planned review: August 15

____
Parent's Signature   Date

____
Service Coordinator's Signature   Date

Index